Preparing for the

ARMY COMBAT FITNESS TEST

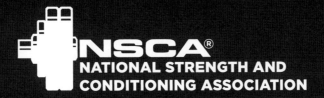

NSCA®
NATIONAL STRENGTH AND
CONDITIONING ASSOCIATION

Nate Palin, MS, CSCS

Rob Hartman, MAEd, CSCS

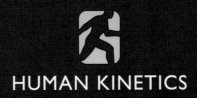

HUMAN KINETICS

Library of Congress Cataloging-in-Publication Data

Names: Palin, Nate, 1980- author. | Hartman, Rob, 1980- author. | National
  Strength & Conditioning Association (U.S.), sponsoring body.
Title: Preparing for the Army Combat Fitness Test / Nate Palin, Rob
  Hartman.
Description: Champaign, IL : Human Kinetics, 2021. | Includes
  bibliographical references.
Identifiers: LCCN 2020016345 (print) | LCCN 2020016346 (ebook) | ISBN
  9781492598688 (paperback) | ISBN 9781492598695 (epub) | ISBN
  9781492598701 (pdf)
Subjects: LCSH: United States. Army--Physical training. | Physical fitness.
  | Exercise.
Classification: LCC U323 .P35 2021 (print) | LCC U323 (ebook) | DDC
  613.7076--dc23
LC record available at https://lccn.loc.gov/2020016345
LC ebook record available at https://lccn.loc.gov/2020016346

ISBN: 978-1-4925-9868-8 (print)

Copyright © 2021 by the National Strength and Conditioning Association

The web addresses cited in this text were current as of March 2020, unless otherwise noted.

Senior Acquisitions Editor: Roger W. Earle; **Developmental Editor:** Amy Stahl; **Copyeditor:** Marissa Wold Uhrina; **Permissions Manager:** Martha Gullo; **Senior Graphic Designer:** Joe Buck; **Cover Designer:** Keri Evans; **Cover Design Specialist:** Susan Rothermel Allen; **Photograph (cover):** Courtesy of the U.S. Army/Capt. Daniel Parker; **Photographs (interior):** © Human Kinetics /Alberto Leopizzi, unless otherwise noted; **Photo Asset Manager:** Laura Fitch; **Photo Production Specialist:** Amy M. Rose; **Photo Production Manager:** Jason Allen; **Senior Art Manager:** Kelly Hendren; **Illustrations:** © Human Kinetics; **Printer:** Walsworth

We thank the National Strength and Conditioning Association in Colorado Springs, Colorado, for providing the location for the photo shoot for this book. We also thank Matthew Sandstead, NSCA-CPT,*D for his assistance in overseeing the photo shoot.

Human Kinetics books are available at special discounts for bulk purchase. Special editions or book excerpts can also be created to specification. For details, contact the Special Sales Manager at Human Kinetics.

Printed in the United States of America

10 9 8 7 6 5 4 3 2 1

The paper in this book was manufactured using responsible forestry methods.

Human Kinetics
1607 N. Market Street
Champaign, IL 61820
USA

United States and International
Website: **US.HumanKinetics.com**
Email: info@hkusa.com
Phone: 1-800-747-4457

Canada
Website: **Canada.HumanKinetics.com**
Email: info@hkcanada.com

E8088

Tell us what you think!
Human Kinetics would love to hear what we
can do to improve the customer experience.
Use this QR code to take our brief survey.

Preparing for the

ARMY COMBAT FITNESS TEST

CONTENTS

Part IV Workout and Exercise Descriptions 137

INTRODUCTION

SUMMARY OF HOW TO USE THIS BOOK

The arrival of the Army Combat Fitness Test (ACFT) causes concern within Army leadership and subordinate soldiers alike because passing the new test requires a more advanced training approach than its Army Physical Fitness Test (APFT) predecessor. Commonly expressed concerns include passing rates (particularly for female soldiers), logistics of training and testing, and potential for injury. The *FM 7-22: Army Physical Readiness Training* field manual (see the web address in the Suggested Resources section of the book) provides leaders with guidance on how to train physically; however, FM 7-22 can be an overwhelming reference that does not effectively communicate a viable training plan to soldiers, particularly with the desired result of passing the ACFT. To bridge the divide left by FM 7-22, this book serves as a comprehensive training guide for both soldiers looking to individually improve their scores and leaders responsible for preparing their soldiers to pass the ACFT.

There is no substitute for direct engagement with a certified strength and conditioning coach. However, *Preparing for the Army Combat Fitness Test* provides a viable solution by describing the ACFT in detail, advising how to evaluate and interpret your results, and providing comprehensive training programs to improve your performance outcomes. An extensive section explains how to safely and effectively execute the exercises assigned within the training programs. Alternative exercises are identified in case you are training under conditions that are less than ideal. This book serves as a standalone resource to help you effectively increase your ACFT score by enhancing essential components of performance.

To best use this book, invest some time in reading part I to better appreciate the reasons for the development of the ACFT and gain familiarity with its six events. Next, read part II to learn some helpful context regarding the principle-based foundation of an effective preparatory training program. Whether you have already taken a test or not, read the start of part III next to understand how your results influence the focus of your training. The remainder of part III then serves as a guide for selecting the best training program given your logistical advantages and limitations. Once you select the most appropriate plan, part IV is a beneficial reference guide that systematically discusses the focus, setup, execution, and common faults associated with each programmed exercise (see figure I.1). Testing upon completion of your selected program serves as a guide for progressive training and allows you to determine which program fits your newly trained state.

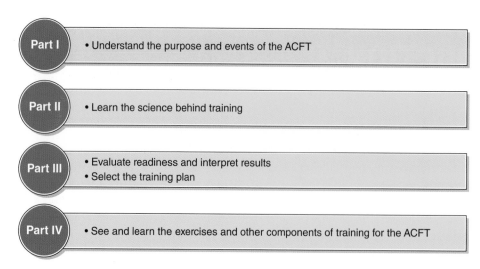

Figure I.1   How to navigate *Preparing for the Army Combat Fitness Test.*

HISTORY OF MILITARY FITNESS TESTING

Before embarking on training for the Army's latest physical fitness test, it helps to understand and appreciate its origins. The Army has a long history of physical testing dating back to the 1850s. The Individual Efficiency Test of 1920 required sprinting, jumping, climbing, throwing, and navigating an obstacle course; furthermore, initial science-based test events in the 1940s consisted of pull-ups, burpees, squat jumps, push-ups, man carries, sit-ups, and a 300-yard (274 m) run.

Ironically, these earlier assessments reflected an appreciation for performing job-relevant activities, a concept aligned with the reemerging trend of functional fitness. Mandatory testing did not occur until the mid-1960s. Shortly thereafter, standardization of the APFT was attempted in an effort to reduce the Army's excessive variety of assessments. Considered less functional by experts in the field of human performance, the APFT was officially incorporated around 1980 as a result of popular American society's shift in fitness trends.

The APFT's commonly known events include two minutes of push-ups, two minutes of sit-ups, and a two-mile run for time, measuring a soldier's ability to perform physically while moving his own body weight. In an analysis of testing results from soldiers dating back to the late 1970s through 2015, researchers found small increases in push-up scores, averaging around low to mid-60s in repetitions, and a similarly small increase in sit-up scores, from mid-sixties to high 60s or low 70s. They also saw a decrease in 2-mile run performance, from low 13-minutes to mid-14-minutes, as well as an increase in both body weight and body mass index (BMI). These results suggest little change to average scores over the last three decades. In the Army, physical fitness tests are the primary driver of physical training; therefore, the Army recognized a need to upgrade its test to influence an increase in the physical abilities and combat readiness of its soldiers.

The APFT that dominated almost 40 years of the Army's physical testing received immense criticism because it focused on muscular and aerobic endurance. The problem with this approach is that it ignored the contributions of strength, power, and movement variability necessary to perform soldiering tasks. Special operations forces (SOF) seemed to acknowledge the APFT's shortcomings; their selection processes typically included additional test events such as maximum repetition pull-ups, foot marching set distances under load for time, obstacle courses, and water survival assessments. Likewise, strength and conditioning coaches within SOF have been administering broader physical assessments that provide a more well-rounded overview of an operator's physicality. The Ranger Regiment's Ranger Athlete Warrior (RAW) assessment includes 10 different events, while the most current initiative, Special Operations Human Performance and Wellness (formerly Preservation of the Force and Family [POTFF]), includes five events. The events include the overhead squat for assessing dynamic mobility and stability, broad jump for assessing power, 5-10-5 drill for agility, trap bar deadlift for lower-body strength, and the 300-meter (328 yd) shuttle for assessing anaerobic endurance. These five events, especially when combined with the APFT, provide coaches with a profile for each soldier that enables more targeted programming to develop physical traits that relate strongly to the demands of the battlefield. The ACFT aims to achieve a similar result. That said, let's look at the Army's newest physical fitness test.

BRIEF DESCRIPTION OF THE ARMY COMBAT FITNESS TEST

Soldiers operate on a three-dimensional battlefield where physical demands are often variable and unpredictable. The Army examined several common soldiering tasks and determined that their completion requires 10 different components of fitness. (This book simplifies the Army's extensive list down to 7 components of performance.) As a result, the muscular- and aerobic endurance-biased APFT gives way to this new test that provides a more diverse measurement of a soldier's physical abilities. The new ACFT is a six-event assessment of physical qualities researched and validated as relevant to common soldiering tasks. Successfully passing the events is intended to demonstrate a modernized physical emphasis that reduces risk of injury, enhances unit readiness, and evolves the Army's physical culture in a way that positively influences mental toughness.

The events include the 3 Repetition Maximum Deadlift (MDL), Standing Power Throw (SPT), Hand Release Push-Up–Arm Extension (HRP), Sprint-Drag-Carry (SDC), Leg Tuck (LTK), and Two-Mile Run (2MR)—performed in that order (figure I.2).

In appreciation for the differing degrees of physicality needed to adequately support various military occupational specialties (MOS), minimum scoring standards are tiered in three levels: jobs with high physical demand, significant physical demand, and moderate physical demand.

The raw physical characteristics tested by the new battery of events include strength, power, muscular endurance, anaerobic endurance, speed, agility, and aerobic endurance. While not tested directly, achieving a passing score on each of six successive events that tax the soldier's entire system requires work capacity and movement competency. The ACFT is discussed in detail in the first seven chapters of the book.

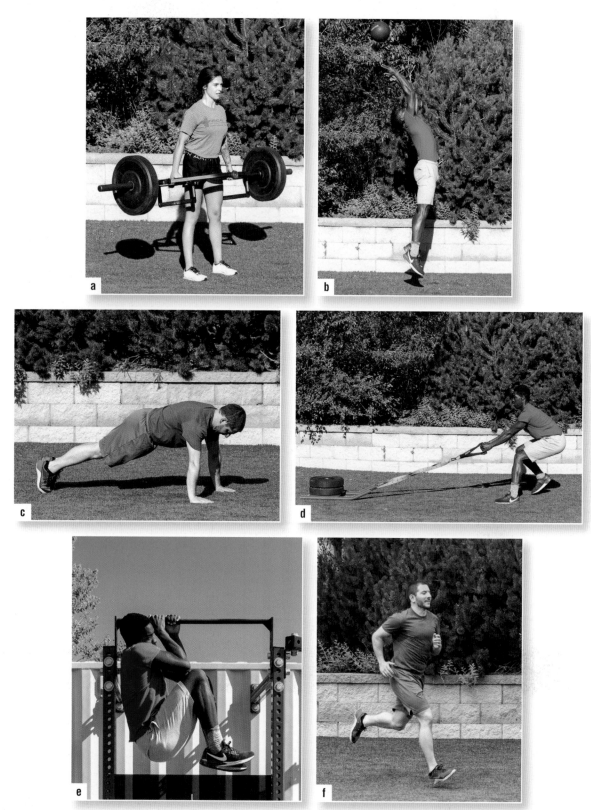

Figure I.2 Examples of the ACFT events: *(a)* 3 Repetition Maximum Deadlift, *(b)* Standing Power Throw, *(c)* Hand Release Push-Up–Arm Extension, *(d)* Sprint-Drag-Carry, *(e)* Leg Tuck, and *(f)* Two-Mile Run.

PART

I

All About the ACFT

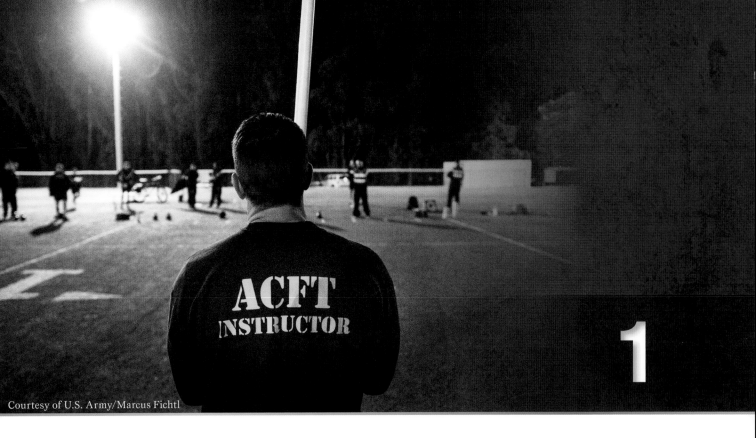

1

The Army Combat Fitness Test

PURPOSE

The Army recognizes that its former Army Physical Fitness Test (APFT) did not drive the best training practices to support mission success. As a result, it invested countless time and resources into developing a new test that requires a type and level of physicality similar to what is needed to perform common soldiering tasks. According to www.army.ml/acft, the Army Combat Fitness Test (ACFT) is intended to "better connect fitness with combat readiness for all soldiers" by achieving the following four outcomes:

1. Improve soldier and unit readiness
2. Transform the Army's fitness culture
3. Reduce preventable injuries and attrition
4. Enhance mental toughness and stamina

To successfully achieve these outcomes and fulfill the intended purpose of the ACFT, the Army's physical training approach requires an upgrade from its tradition of push-ups, sit-ups, and distance running. Implementing a new test with pass-or-fail implications prior to providing appropriate training strategies can increase injury risk during both training and testing and is also likely to result in a failure rate that exposes shortcomings in the Army's approach to fitness. However, assuming necessary adjustments are continuously incorporated within physical training, the ACFT should eventually achieve its purpose.

WHAT TO EXPECT

You can expect a longer and logistically intensive test that requires a comprehensive display of physicality to successfully pass. It will be hard to hide your physical weaknesses because so many performance traits are tested by the six events (discussed in detail in the next six chapters). Excelling on the ACFT requires power, strength, and endurance, all built on a foundation of movement competency. These are the same underlying physical characteristics that likely support success in your unit's mission essential task listings (METL). Training to improve performance on the test and training to improve job performance now have a high level of compatibility compared to the one-dimensional APFT. Aerobic and muscular endurance are still essential qualities for passing, but the ACFT requires increased focus on other components of well-rounded athleticism.

Logistically, the ACFT requires a lot of time, equipment, space, and manpower. The test must be completed within 90 minutes; however, according to the Army's Quick Reference Guide, most participants will finish in less than 75 minutes. A 5-minute rest period is allowed between all tests, and a 10-minute rest period is allowed prior to starting the last event, which is the two-mile run. For equipment, the ACFT requires a 60-pound (27 kg) trap bar and bumper plates, a 10-pound (5 kg) medicine ball, two 40-pound (18 kg) kettlebells, a 90-pound (41 kg) sled with straps for pulling, and a pull-up bar per lane (figure 1.1).

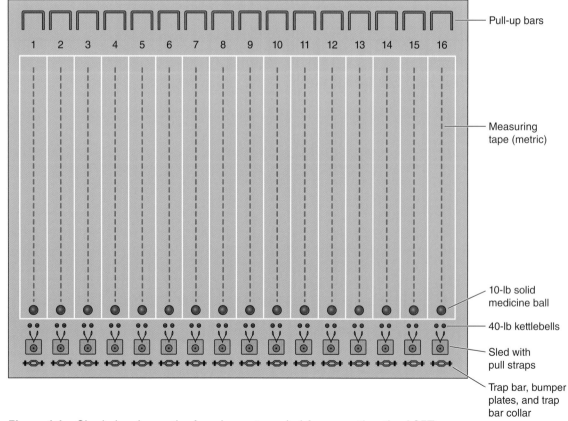

Figure 1.1   Single lane's worth of equipment needed for executing the ACFT.

Recommended grading equipment includes stopwatches, 25-meter (27 yd) tape measures, sticks to mark the Standing Power Throw (SPT), tall traffic cones, and small field cones. Each unit should possess its own standardized locker full of the necessary testing equipment. The test also requires open space with enough width and length to accommodate the SPT and Sprint-Drag-Carry (SDC) events, and a level, improved running service totaling two miles. Either a Non-Commissioned Officer or an Officer in Charge oversees the test's administration, and a certified ACFT grader is required for each lane (two to four soldiers perform the events within each lane). The number of lanes depends on the size of the unit and space available for each event. The next six chapters explain execution and scoring of each of the six ACFT events.

SCORING STANDARDS

As discussed in the introduction, ACFT scoring standards vary based on military occupational specialties (MOS). Table 1.1 depicts minimum passing scores for each event based on physical categorization of each MOS and criteria for maximum potential score per event.

The moderate (or "gold") minimum passing score is 60 points on each event. As of the date of publication, due to training disruptions caused by the international coronavirus pandemic, the Army is opting to hold every MOS category to achieving the moderate minimum passing score of 60 points on each event. ACFT scores will not be used administratively for punitive reasons and promotion-related purposes until March 2022. ACFT scores will be recorded as a test of record, but it is the soldier's last APFT of record that counts for the administrative purposes previously mentioned and for admission to military schools.

Table 1.1   ACFT Scoring Standards

Points	MDL (Pounds)	SPT (Meters)	HRP (Repetitions)	SDC (Time)	LTK (Repetitions)	2MR (Time)	
100	340	12.5	60	1:33	20	13:30	All MAX
99		12.4	59	1:36		13:39	
98		12.2	58	1:39	19	13:48	
97	330	12.1	57	1:41		13:57	
96		11.9	56	1:43	18	14:06	
95		11.8	55	1:45		14:15	
94	320	11.6	54	1:46	17	14:24	
93		11.5	53	1:47		14:33	
92	310	11.3	52	1:48	16	14:42	
91		11.2	51	1:49		14:51	
90	300	11.0	50	1:50	15	15:00	
89		10.9	49	1:51		15:09	
88	290	10.7	48	1:52	14	15:18	
87		10.6	47	1:53		15:27	
86	280	10.4	46	1:54	13	15:36	
85		10.3	45	1:55		15:45	
84	270	10.1	44	1:56	12	15:54	
83		10.0	43	1:57		16:03	
82	260	9.8	42	1:58	11	16:12	
81		9.7	41	1:59		16:21	
80	250	9.5	40	2:00	10	16:30	
79		9.4	39	2:01		16:39	
78	240	9.2	38	2:02	9	16:48	
77		9.1	37	2:03		16:57	
76	230	8.9	36	2:04	8	17:06	
75		8.8	35	2:05		17:15	
74	220	8.6	34	2:06	7	17:24	
73		8.5	33	2:07		17:33	
72	210	8.3	32	2:08	6	17:42	
71		8.2	31	2:09		17:51	
70	200	8.0	30	2:10	5	18:00	Heavy MIN
69		7.8	28	2:14		18:12	
68	190	7.5	26	2:18	4	18:24	
67		7.1	24	2:22		18:36	
66		6.8	22	2:26		18:48	

Points	MDL (Pounds)	SPT (Meters)	HRP (Repetitions)	SDC (Time)	LTK (Repetitions)	2MR (Time)	
65	180	6.5	20	2:30	3	19:00	Significant MIN
64	170	6.2	18	2:35		19:24	
63	160	5.8	16	2:40		19:48	
62	150	5.4	14	2:45	2	20:12	
61		4.9	12	2:50		20:36	
60	140	4.5	10	3:00	1*	21:00	Moderate MIN
59				3:01		21:01	
58				3:02		21:03	
57				3:03		21:05	
56				3:04		21:07	
55		4.4	9	3:05		21:09	
54				3:06		21:10	
53				3:07		21:12	
52				3:08		21:14	
51				3:09		21:16	
50	130	4.3	8	3:10		21:18	
49						21:19	
48				3:11		21:21	
47						21:23	
46				3:12		21:25	
45		4.2	7			21:27	
44				3:13		21:28	
43						21:30	
42				3:14		21:32	
41						21:34	
40	120	4.1	6	3:15		21:36	
39						21:37	
38				3:16		21:39	
37						21:41	
36				3:17		21:43	
35		4.0	5			21:45	
34				3:18		21:46	
33						21:48	
32				3:19		21:50	
31						21:52	
30	110	3.9	4	3:20		21:54	
29						21:55	
28				3:21		21:57	

(continued)

Table 1.1   *(continued)*

Points	MDL (Pounds)	SPT (Meters)	HRP (Repetitions)	SDC (Time)	LTK (Repetitions)	2MR (Time)	
27						21:59	
26				3:22		22:01	
25		3.8	3			22:03	
24				3:23		22:04	
23						22:06	
22				3:24		22:08	
21						22:10	
20	100	3.7	2	3:25		22:12	
19						22:13	
18				3:26		22:15	
17						22:17	
16				3:27		22:19	
15		3.6	1			22:21	
14				3:28		22:22	
13						22:24	
12				3:29		22:26	
11						22:28	
10	90	3.5		3:30		22:30	
9						22:31	
8				3:31		22:33	
7						22:35	
6				3:32		22:37	
5		3.4				22:39	
4				3:33		22:40	
3						22:42	
2				3:34		22:44	
1						22:46	
0	80	3.3	0	3:35		22:48	

As of October 1, 2019.

1 pound = 0.45 kilogram

1 meter = 1.1 yard

MDL = 3 Repetition Maximum Deadlift; SPT = Standing Power Throw; HRP = Hand Release Push-Up–Arm Extension, SDC = Sprint-Drag-Carry; LTK = Leg Tuck; 2MR = Two-Mile Run

* 2:00 for alternative Plank event if soldier fails the Leg Tuck

Reprinted from Appendix 3 to Annex A, HQDA EXORD 219-18, https://www.army.mil/acft (March 24, 2020).

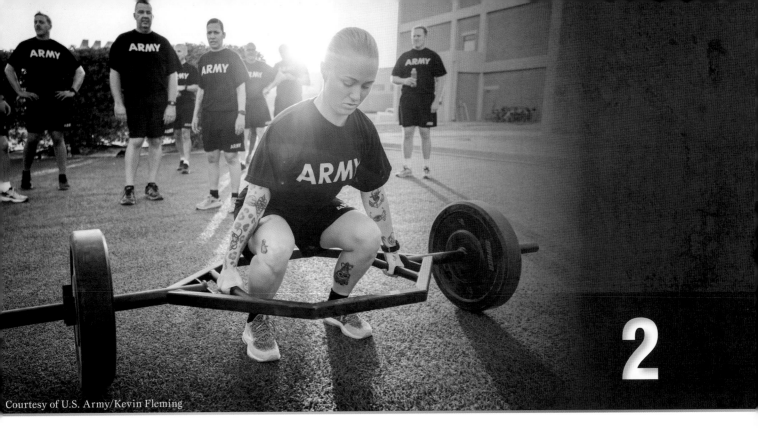

2

3 Repetition Maximum Deadlift

The 3 Repetition Maximum Deadlift (MDL) assesses lower-body pulling combined with pushing, grip, and isometric back strength. These are undeniably essential components of countless soldiering tasks such as movement under fire and under load, evacuating a casualty from a vehicle or threat, and moving or loading heavy ammunition containers. The test uses a standardized 60-pound (27 kg) trap bar with bumper plates. If a dual-handled trap bar is used, the lower handles must be used with the higher handles facing down.

Beginning from a dead stop (figure 2.1), the weight must be moved from the ground to a full standing position without compromising the soldier's back position. The standing, or lockout, position consists of fully extended knees and hips (figure 2.2). The weight must be returned to the ground under control. These actions are repeated three times with the maximum weight possible.

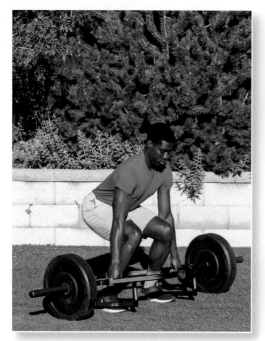 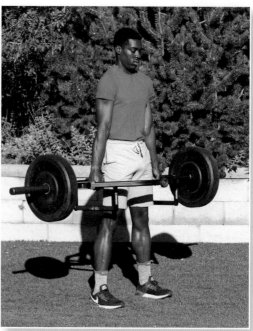

Figure 2.1   3 Repetition Maximum Deadlift: beginning or dead stop (bottom) position.

Figure 2.2   3 Repetition Maximum Deadlift: ending or lockout (top) position.

SCORING STANDARDS

Every repetition must start from a dead stop; bouncing off the floor between repetitions is not permitted. If three successful repetitions are performed at the attempted weight, a heavier triple can be attempted. Likewise, if all three repetitions are not successfully completed, a lighter weight can be attempted after a rest of two minutes. Note that only two total test sets are permitted. Failure to achieve three repetitions on both test sets results in a score of 0 and failure of the ACFT. Soldiers are encouraged to perform their first test set at their MOS minimum. Starting with a higher weight is permitted, but it increases the risk of not receiving a passing score on the MDL. Additional warmup sets are not permitted currently between the first and second test attempt. Soldiers who open with a safe weight typically make a massive jump on their second attempt, while soldiers who open with an aggressive weight tend to drop to their MOS minimum to ensure a passing score.

A maximum score of 100 is earned by deadlifting 340 pounds (155 kg) for three repetitions. Table 2.1 shows the minimum scores for each type of MOS.

Table 2.1   3 Repetition Maximum Deadlift Scoring Minimums per MOS Category

Moderate (60 points)	Significant (65 points)	Heavy (70 points)
140 pounds	180 pounds	200 pounds

As of October 1, 2019.

1 pound = 0.45 kilogram

Reprinted from Appendix 3 to Annex A, HQDA EXORD 219-18, https://www.army.mil/acft (March 24, 2020).

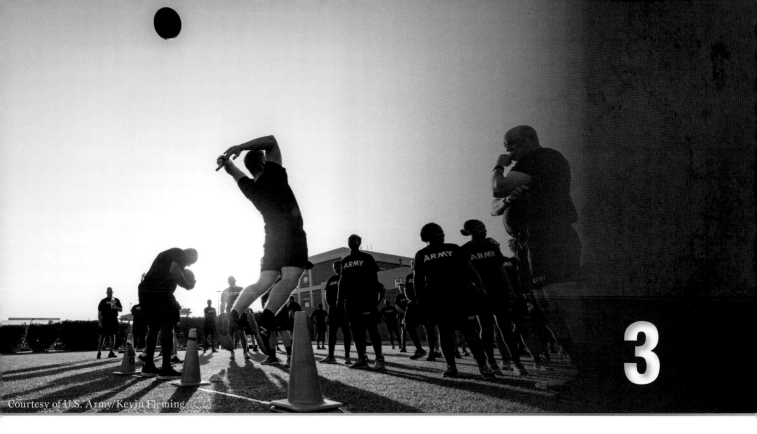

Courtesy of U.S. Army/Kevin Fleming

3

Standing Power Throw

The Standing Power Throw (SPT) assesses total body explosiveness in appreciation for the role of **power** in countless soldiering tasks such as traversing uneven terrain, jumping, grenade throwing, operating in urban environments (especially breaching), and moving equipment over barriers. While it reigns supreme in athletic culture, power is a traditionally underappreciated and, therefore, undertrained component of performance within the Army.

The SPT event uses a 10-pound (5 kg) medicine ball. Starting with your heels in contact with the ground behind the line and the ball at hip height, you can bend your hips, knees, and ankles in preparation for launching the ball backward and overhead (figure 3.1). Triple extension of the ankles, knees, and hips is allowed, as is leaving the ground (figure 3.2), so long as no part of the body crosses the line. The feet or any part of the body crossing the line results in a fault.

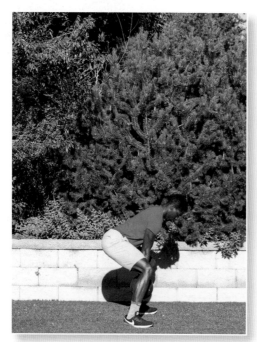 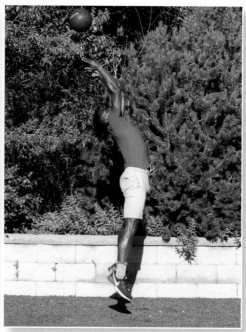

Figure 3.1   Standing Power Throw: beginning (flexed) position.

Figure 3.2   Standing Power Throw: ending (extended) position.

SCORING STANDARDS

Three total throws are allowed but only if the first two result in consecutive faults. Otherwise, a nonfaulted score within your first two attempts counts and only the furthest throw counts toward your score. The maximum achievable score of 100 is earned by throwing the medicine ball 12.5 meters (13.7 yd). Table 3.1 shows the minimum scores for each type of MOS.

Table 3.1   Standing Power Throw Scoring Minimums per MOS Category

Moderate (60 points)	Significant (65 points)	Heavy (70 points)
4.5 meters	6.5 meters	8.0 meters

As of October 1, 2019.

1 meter = 1.1 yard

Reprinted from Appendix 3 to Annex A, HQDA EXORD 219-18, https://www.army.mil/acft (March 24, 2020).

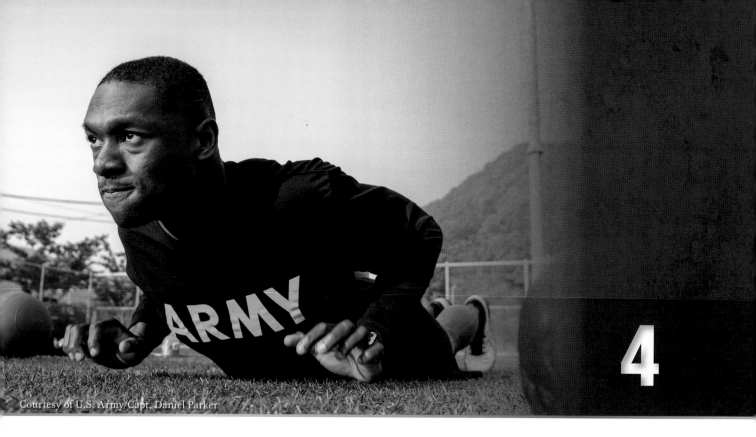

4

Hand Release Push-Up–Arm Extension

The Hand Release Push-Up–Arm Extension (HRP) tests upper-body pushing endurance, possibly an overemphasized physical characteristic that is less directly relatable to soldiering tasks. However, it is still applicable to movement under fire and hand-to-hand combat. The event also requires a substantial amount of upper-body flexibility to minimize risk of injury during testing.

While you might be familiar with the push-up test from the APFT, the HRP is unique. You must start from a prone position with your chest, hips, and thighs (but not head) in contact with the ground and index fingers inside the broadest part of your shoulders (figure 4.1). Maintaining a fairly straight line from the head to the heel, and the feet no more than a boot's width apart, push yourself up until your arms are fully extended (figure 4.2). When lowering down, the same three points of contact (chest, hips, and thighs) should touch the ground in unison (figure 4.3). Once back in the prone position, extend your arms directly out to your sides, forming a T (figure 4.4). Bring the hands back under the shoulders, place them on the ground, then lift them up again to start the next repetition.

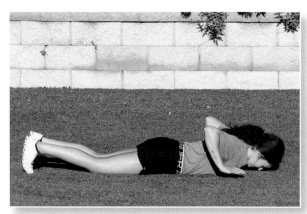

Figure 4.1   Hand Release Push-Up–Arm Extension: beginning position.

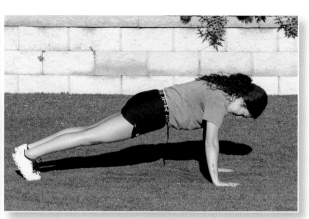

Figure 4.2   Hand Release Push-Up–Arm Extension: up position.

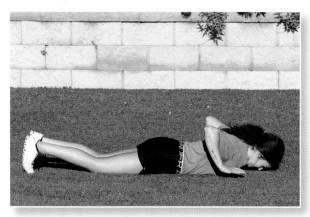

Figure 4.3   Hand Release Push-Up–Arm Extension: return to ground.

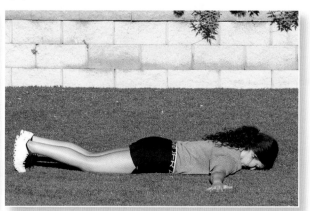

Figure 4.4   Hand Release Push-Up–Arm Extension: arms extended in T position.

SCORING STANDARDS

Notably, no authorized rest position exists except the top position where the arms are extended and the body is straight. You cannot rest on the ground nor can you rest in positions common to the APFT's push-up event; lack of continuous effort results in termination of the event. The maximum achievable score of 100 is earned by completing 60 repetitions. Table 4.1 shows the minimum scores for each type of MOS.

Table 4.1   Hand Release Push-Up–Arm Extension Scoring Minimums per MOS Category

Moderate (60 points)	Significant (65 points)	Heavy (70 points)
10 repetitions	20 repetitions	30 repetitions

As of October 1, 2019.

Reprinted from Appendix 3 to Annex A, HQDA EXORD 219-18, https://www.army.mil/acft (March 24, 2020).

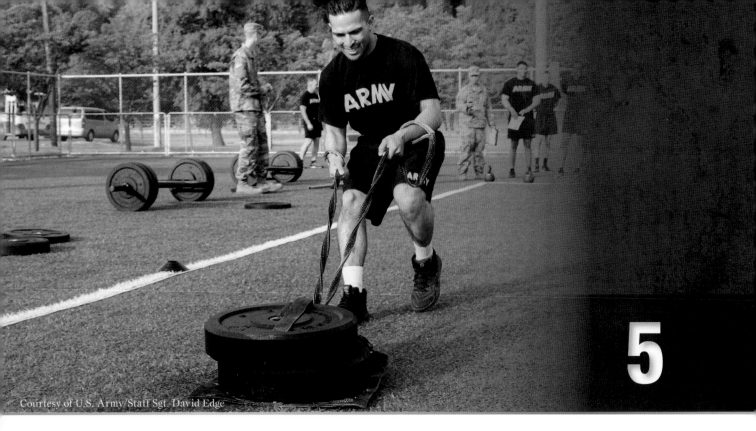
Courtesy of U.S. Army/Staff Sgt. David Edge

5

Sprint-Drag-Carry

The Sprint-Drag-Carry (SDC) event tests primarily anaerobic capacity with components of lower- and upper-body strength and muscular endurance. Relevant soldiering tasks include evacuating a casualty, ammunition resupply, movement under fire and during urban operations, breaking contact, and mountaineering. The test requires two 40-pound (18 kg) kettlebells and a 90-pound (41 kg) sled. You must complete five shuttles of 25 meters (27 yd) in each direction while performing a sprint for the first, sled drag for the second, lateral shuffle for the third, kettlebell carry for the fourth, and another sprint for the fifth (figure 5.1).

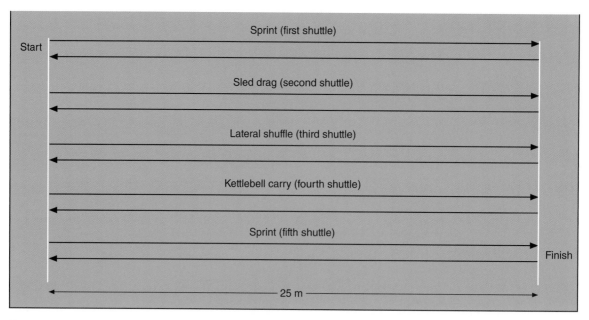

Figure 5.1   Sprint-Drag-Carry: overview diagram.

The beginning position for the event consists of a prone position with the entire body (including the head) behind the start line (figure 5.2). For the sprints (figure 5.3), you must touch the 25-meter (27 yd) line with both your foot and your hand. For the drag, the sled must be pulled backward until the entire sled crosses the 25-meter (27 yd) line and pulled backward back to the start until the entire sled crosses the start line (figure 5.4). For the lateral shuffle, you must remain sideways without crossing the feet (figure 5.5), and you must touch the 25-meter (27 yd) line with both a hand and foot. For the carry, you must touch the 25-meter line (27 yd) (or beyond it) with one foot (figure 5.6). The carry portion concludes when the kettlebells are set down at the start (after stepping on or beyond the line) and the final sprint begins. Once again, the 25-meter (27 yd) line must be touched with both a hand and foot, and the test concludes when you sprint through the start line (figure 5.7).

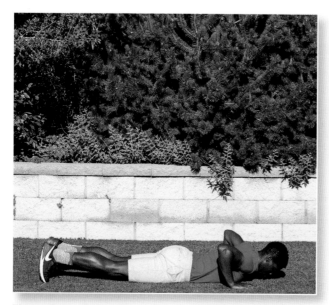

Figure 5.2   Sprint-Drag-Carry: beginning (prone) position.

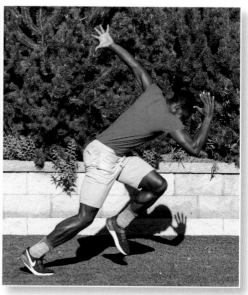

Figure 5.3   Sprint-Drag-Carry: acceleration.

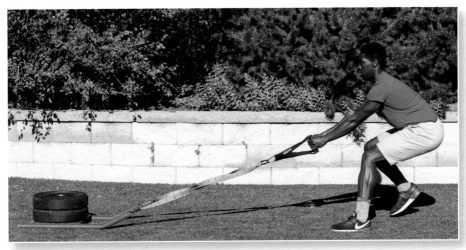

Figure 5.4 Sprint-Drag-Carry: sled drag.

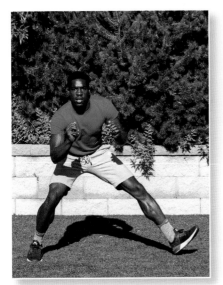

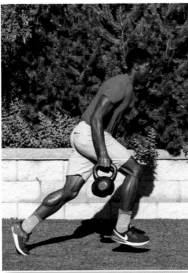

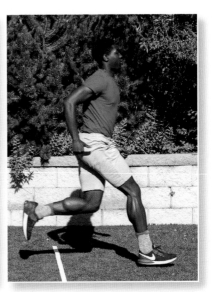

Figure 5.5 Sprint-Drag-Carry: lateral shuffle.

Figure 5.6 Sprint-Drag-Carry: kettlebell carry.

Figure 5.7 Sprint-Drag-Carry: sprint (crossing finish line).

SCORING STANDARDS

The maximum achievable score of 100 is earned by completing all five laps in 1 minute and 33 seconds or less. Table 5.1 shows the minimum scores for each type of MOS.

Table 5.1 Sprint-Drag-Carry Scoring Minimums per MOS Category

Moderate (60 points)	Significant (65 points)	Heavy (70 points)
3:00	2:30	2:10

As of October 1, 2019.

Min:sec

Reprinted from Appendix 3 to Annex A, HQDA EXORD 219-18, https://www.army.mil/acft (March 24, 2020).

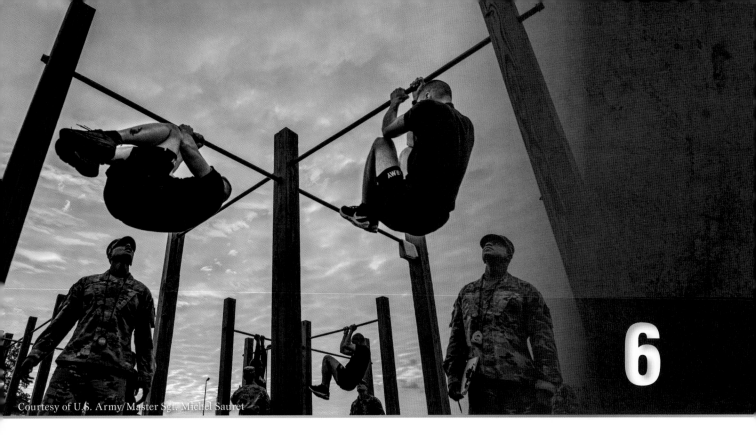

6

Leg Tuck

The Leg Tuck (LTK) event tests strength and endurance of the abdominals and hip flexors, arms, upper back, and grip. In the experience of Major Donny Bigham, head strength coach at the Army's Tactical Athlete Performance Center (TAP-C), grip reflects the biggest determinant for success on the LTK. He recommends that the baseline grip strength of both hands combined (as measured by a dynamometer) should equal the weight of the soldier while wearing personal protection equipment.

The only equipment needed for the LTK is a pull-up bar. Relevant soldiering tasks include any that involve climbing or require anterior core strength, like combatives and shooting from various positions.

The test starts from a dead hang position with straight arms and an alternated grip on the bar (figure 6.1). To execute the LTK action, bend your arms at the elbows and bring your knees or thighs up to touch your elbows before returning to the beginning position (figure 6.2).

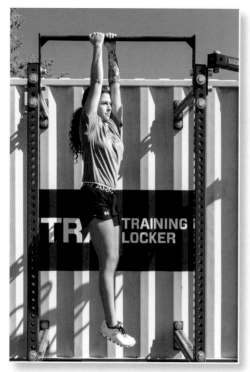

Figure 6.1   Leg Tuck: beginning position.

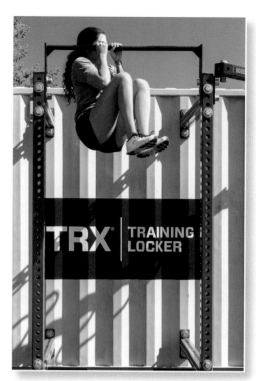

Figure 6.2   Leg Tuck: ending position.

SCORING STANDARDS

The test allows for some minor movements in the dead hang position but intentional swinging to assist in bringing the knees up is not allowed. Grip adjustments are permitted as long as you do not drop to the ground. The maximum achievable score of 100 is achieved by completing 20 consecutive LTKs. Table 6.1 shows the minimum score for each type of MOS.

Table 6.1   **Leg Tuck Scoring Minimums per MOS Category**

Moderate (60 points)	Significant (65 points)	Heavy (70 points)
1 repetition	3 repetitions	5 repetitions

As of October 1, 2019.

Reprinted from Appendix 3 to Annex A, HQDA EXORD 219-18, https://www.army.mil/acft (March 24, 2020).

INTERIM ALTERNATIVE EVENT

To facilitate a successful transition to the Leg Tuck event, the Army is allowing the completion of a two-minute Plank as a means of earning a passing score of 60 points for soldiers who attempt and fail to execute a single Leg Tuck. Proper Plank execution consists of holding a position with the elbows directly under the shoulders, setting up the feet the same as the Hand Release Push-Up—Arm Extension, and maintaining a fairly straight line from the top of the head through the heel of the foot (figure 6.3). The maximum achievable score for the Plank alternative is 60 points, and failure to perform a two-minute Plank results in a score of 0 for the Leg Tuck event. The Plank is only offered as an alternative for an interim period of time, and soldiers should focus on passing the Leg Tuck event based on primary scoring standards.

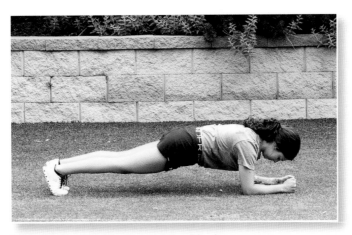

Figure 6.3   Lateral view of the Plank.

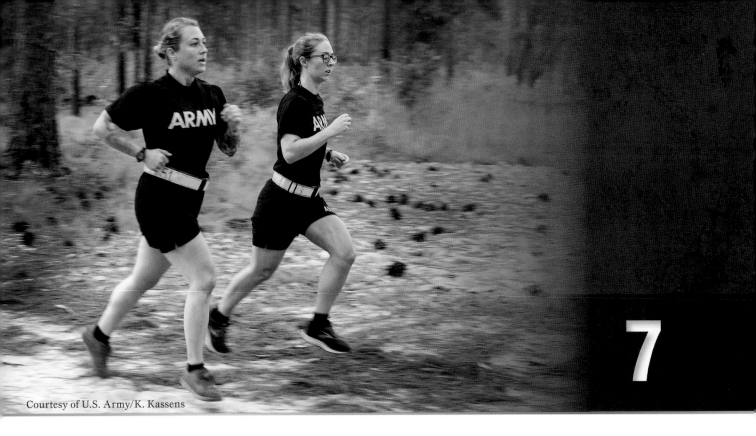

Courtesy of U.S. Army/K. Kassens

7

Two-Mile Run

The Two-Mile Run (2MR) is the only event carried over from the APFT; however, the scoring standards have changed because it is preceded by several physically-demanding events that result in starting the run in a more prefatigued state.

The event tests aerobic endurance with a specific appreciation for the skill of running. Aerobic endurance is an essential component of performance that contributes to soldiering tasks such as ruck marching, land navigation, recovery between higher-intensity activities, and even general cardiovascular health. The only equipment needed is running shoes along with access to a relatively flat two-mile course (no unimproved terrain is allowed, but the course can be one mile out and back) (figure 7.1). The test consists of a timed two-mile run conducted five minutes after the final soldier completes the LTK.

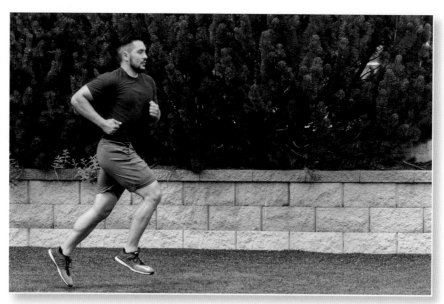

Figure 7.1   The Two-Mile Run.

SCORING STANDARDS

The maximum achievable score of 100 is achieved by completing the 2MR in 13:30 or less. Table 7.1 shows the minimum score for each type of MOS.

Table 7.1   **Two-Mile Run Scoring Minimums per MOS Category**

Moderate (60 points)	Significant (65 points)	Heavy (70 points)
21:00	19:00	18:00

As of October 1, 2019.

Min:sec

Reprinted from Appendix 3 to Annex A, HQDA EXORD 219-18, https://www.army.mil/acft (March 24, 2020).

ALTERNATIVE EVENTS

Soldiers who cannot run due to being placed on a medical profile can select one of three alternative aerobic events. These 2MR alternatives are the 1,000-meter swim, 5,000-meter row, and the 12,000-meter stationary cycle (figure 7.2). The alternative event should start within 10 minutes of completing the SDC. To pass, the selected event must be completed within 25 minutes. Stationary bike resistance should be set in the middle, between the highest and lowest resistances possible. Rowing machine resistance is at the discretion of the soldier. Resting is authorized during each event, but the soldier cannot dismount the bike or rowing machine at any point. During the swim, soldiers may rest by standing on the bottom or holding onto the sides of the pool; however, they cannot walk along the bottom. Goggles and a swim cap are authorized.

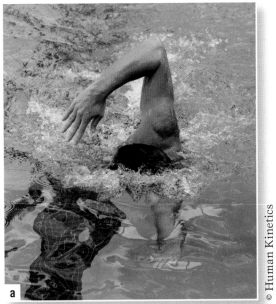

© Human Kinetics

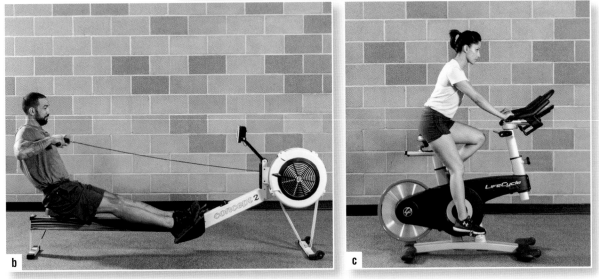

Figure 7.2   Alternative events for the Two-Mile Run are *(a)* the 1,000-meter swim, *(b)* the 5,000-meter row, and *(c)* the 12,000-meter stationary cycle.

The Science Behind Training

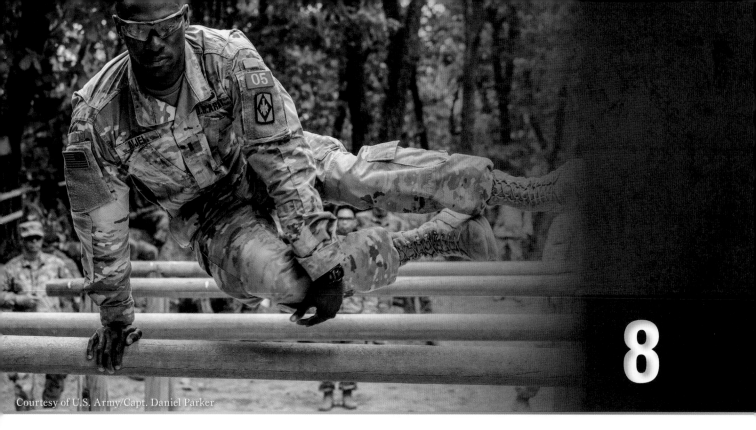

8

Training Principles

INDIVIDUALITY

Every soldier has strengths and weaknesses with regards to physicality. The differences in physical abilities can be attributed to several factors that comprise your individuality. Genetics are an undeniable contributor to your physical ability. Consider an elite sprinter versus an equally elite marathon runner. Each can train to move the needle toward the other's attributes but will never fully close the gap due to genetic differences. Other determinants include age, training experience, injury history, and sex. If **individuality** did not exist, all soldiers would exit Basic Training as physical clones of one another.

Training programs found in chapter 12 are limited in how much they take into account your individuality. However, adjusting exercise selection and intensities to align with individual ability provides some individuality within a generic training program. While a higher level of individuality can be achieved with in-person coaching that includes questionnaires and assessments, chapter 10 (Your Current State of Readiness) provides a self-evaluation and guidance on interpreting your results to help you select the performance components to emphasize in your training.

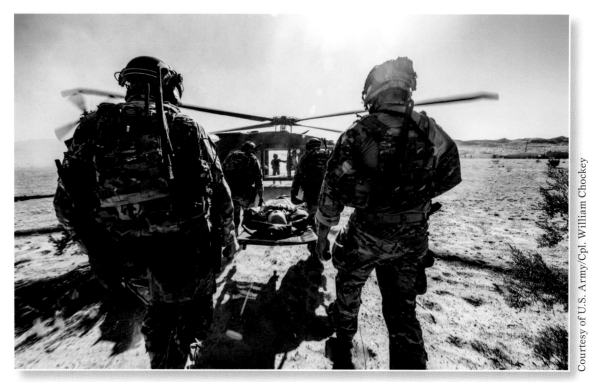

Courtesy of U.S. Army/Cpl. William Chockey

Soldiers complete tasks that require various ranges of motion, movement planes, and energy demands.

SPECIFICITY

Specificity is the principle of targeting physical characteristics related to the successful execution of your job. The body responds directly to the stimulus you provide it, with regards to movement, muscle, and metabolic demands. The reason the ACFT is replacing the APFT is to assist commanders' and soldiers' combat readiness by increasing the specificity of training for a test that better emphasizes performance traits that are relevant to soldiering. Ideal training programs typically compare the athlete's ability against the demands of the sport, then target what is needed to close the gap between them. The same approach works for you as a soldier. Too often, however, specificity is trained with little to no regard for individuality. This can lead at best to an insufficient training stimulus that does not improve physicality, and at worst to an inappropriate stimulus that leads to injury.

Specificity does have its limitations. Consider this: Preparing physically for the demands of being an infantryman does not get more specific than performing the METL or warrior tasks and battle drills (WTBD) of an infantryman. If extremely specific specificity is all that is needed to physically prepare for being an infantryman, there is no need for other physical training. The term *relevance* can sometimes be more appropriate. For example, increasing leg strength with heavy squatting is extremely relevant to the METL of an infantry soldier but it is not as specific as rucking. Relevant training can target underlying physical characteristics that positively affect specific tasks. Rucking does not necessitate leg strength as much as squatting, but squatting can undeniably improve the performance of rucking. Intensity, duration, and planes of movement are all important considerations for achieving relevance in training. Breaching a door is a rotational task that occurs in less than 10 seconds; therefore, training short bursts of rotational power using exercises such as medicine ball throws relates directly to breaching (table 8.1).

Table 8.1   Soldiering Tasks and Corresponding Exercise Examples

Task	Exercise	Movement plane	Energy demand	Performance component
Mechanical door breach	Landmine twist	Transverse	Short duration, high intensity	Power
Lifting a casualty	Deadlift	Sagittal	Short duration, high intensity	Muscular strength
React to contact	Shuttle sprints	Sagittal	Short duration, high intensity	Power, anaerobic endurance
Loading a truck	Shoulder press	Sagittal	Long duration, low intensity	Muscular endurance
Casualty evacuation	Single-arm farmer walk	Frontal	Moderate duration, moderate intensity	Anaerobic and muscular endurance
Offset infiltration	Rucking	Sagittal	Long duration, low intensity	Aerobic endurance

OVERLOAD

When selecting exercise variables such as type, volume, and intensity that are individual to you and specific to the demands of your job, you must sufficiently **overload** them to impose a stimulus strong enough to force your body to adapt favorably. If you can perform 50 unbroken bodyweight push-ups, bodyweight push-ups do not provide enough overload to bring about a change in upper-body strength. Likewise, if you want to run your 2MR faster, only running longer distances at slower speeds might not provide sufficient overload to achieve a decreased 2MR time.

You can overload your body in countless ways. The simplest and arguably the most effective ways to achieve overload are by increasing intensity (speed or resistance) and volume (repetitions, distance, or duration). Increasing complexity can also bring about overload, but simple exercises allow for more competent execution and it is often unnecessary to make them more complicated. If an exercise is too complex, it can be difficult to perform at a sufficient intensity and for a sufficient duration. Keep this in mind when selecting exercises. Overload should be aggressive enough to force favorable change but not so much that it renders you unable to perform the exercise with safe and proper technique. Adjustment of the intensity, volume, or complexity of the exercise provides you a simple but highly effective solution for achieving individuality within a team or unit containing differing physical abilities.

PROGRESSION

A given stimulus might overload you initially, but assuming consistency of training, its effectiveness decreases over time because you have adapted positively to it. This is evidence of positive physical adaptation, the primary reason you applied overload, and signals a need to progress the stimulus to continue to achieve overload. **Progression** is nothing more than the continued application of overload; therefore, this training principle is best executed by increasing intensity, volume, variety, or complexity (table 8.2). Like complexity, variety is a change of stimulus that needs to be applied carefully. If a stimulus changes too frequently, your body does not have time or reason to adapt to it. For this reason, eliminate the socially popular concept of "muscle confusion" from your training plan. Instead, prioritize training consistently (too often the biggest obstacle to progression within the military setting), then look to achieve progression by making minor adjustments in the selection of your stimulus. Regardless of how you adjust

Table 8.2   How to Apply Progression to Various Types of Overload

Type of overload	Progression
Intensity (resistance, speed)	• Increase mechanical disadvantage (change position of the body or resistance to increase difficulty) • Increase intensity (move more weight or move faster)
Volume (distance, duration, repetitions)	• Increase total volume (add repetitions, sets, distance, or duration) • Achieve same volume in less time (i.e., increase density) • Achieve more volume in same time (i.e., increase density)
Complexity	• Increase skill demand • Change force vector (direction from which force is applied relative to the body) or position of load • Add secondary movements • Increase range of motion

training to achieve continuous overload, be sure to provide adequate rest and recovery to allow for positive change to occur. Your body does not adapt during training; it adapts between your training sessions, when proper sleep and nutrition facilitate recovery processes.

Some soldiers progress faster than others. If you are responsible for training other soldiers and cannot individualize their training plans, progress at the pace of your soldier with the slowest advancement. This might not provide sufficient overload to ideally progress the rest of your soldiers but at least reduces the risk of injury and focuses on improving your weakest link.

DIMINISHING RETURNS

Regardless of how intelligently progressive overload is applied, increased exposure to training eventually results in a decrease in your return on investment of both time and effort. Initial increases in physical abilities often arrive rapidly, even without an aggressive stimulus. However, further increases become harder to achieve as your training age increases. Consider how easily you likely improved your physical training (PT) score over the course of Basic Training. Now, try to recall how much more difficult it was to keep increasing your score once you arrived at your unit, particularly when you might not have had access to consistent training or a sufficient stimulus to force change (adaptation).

The closer you are to realizing your genetic potential, the more difficult it will be to obtain impressive performance gains. That said, very few soldiers have undergone consistent enough exposure to proper physical training that their genetic ceiling becomes a barrier to improved performance. Likewise, minimum scoring standards on each event within the ACFT are easily obtainable without implementing extreme performance measures in training.

REVERSIBILITY

Imposing progressive overload consistently with an appreciation for individuality and specificity yields adaptations that enhance physical abilities relevant to the ACFT and your MOS. However, taking time off from training results in detraining due to the principle of reversibility. Simply put—if you do not use it, you lose it. Preventing detraining does not necessitate the volume or frequency of overload required for generating performance improvements; however, applying the same intensity appears necessary to stave off the loss of your hard-earned performance gains. Fortunately, evidence shows that regaining strength is easier than developing it initially.

Different components of performance degrade at different rates (figure 8.1). Speed and power tend to degrade much sooner than strength and aerobic endurance, with anaerobic endurance falling somewhere in the middle. Because of these relative differences in the time it takes to degrade to a detrained state, strength and aerobic capacity can be maintained with minimal effort while you focus on speed, power, and the repeatability of both qualities.

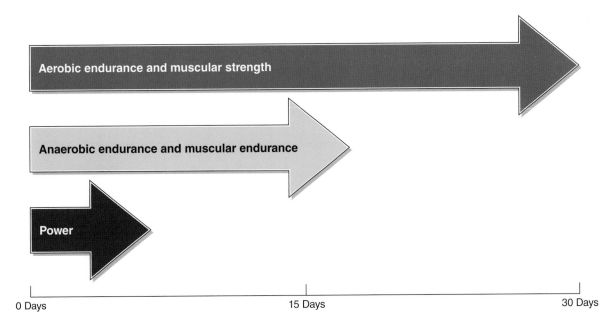

Figure 8.1 Comparative rates of performance component degradation.

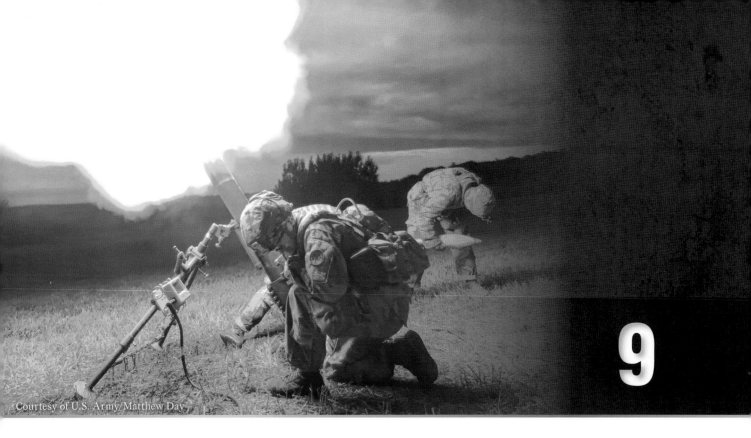

9

Components of Performance

MOVEMENT COMPETENCY

The ability to achieve the positions and rhythms necessary to move efficiently—without compensating or deviating from those efficient movement patterns—is called **movement competency**. Some may think that movement competency is the same thing as flexibility, but movement competency expands to include the interaction of flexibility, mobility, stability, and coordination. Reinforcing dysfunctional movement with strength, power, muscular endurance, and aerobic endurance training can result in acute and chronic injuries that will negatively affect your performance. Contrarily, reinforcing efficient movement with strength, power, muscular endurance, and aerobic endurance can lead to the enhancement of performance. Movement competency is an essential underlying quality of every component: power (to include speed and agility), strength, muscular endurance, and aerobic endurance. It is also essential for the safe, effective, and efficient execution of all six events that comprise the ACFT.

For the sake of simplicity, you need competent movement in the patterns and skills discussed within the exercises programmed in this book:

- Power (figure 9.1a)
- Lower body pulling (figure 9.1b)
- Lower body pushing (figure 9.1c)
- Upper body pulling, both vertically (figure 9.1d) and horizontally (figure 9.1e)
- Upper body pushing, both vertically (figure 9.1f) and horizontally (figure 9.1g)
- Locomotion (mostly found in warmup and conditioning; figures 9.1h-9.1i)
- Trunk actions, such as flexion (figure 9.1j), extension (figure 9.1k), and rotation (figure 9.1l)

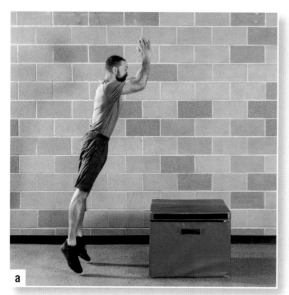

Figure 9.1   *(a)* Power.

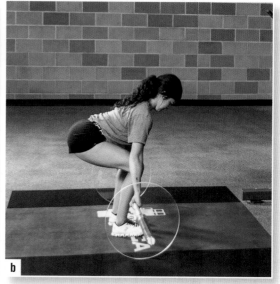

Figure 9.1   *(b)* Lower body pulling.

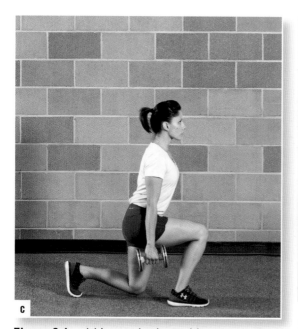

Figure 9.1   *(c)* Lower body pushing.

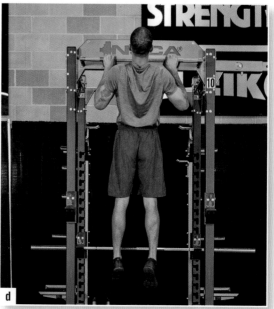

Figure 9.1   *(d)* Upper body pulling, vertically.

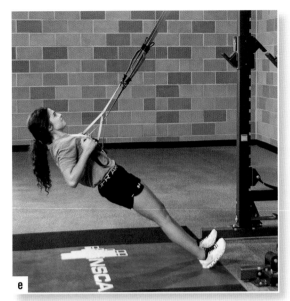

Figure 9.1 *(e)* Upper body pulling, horizontally.

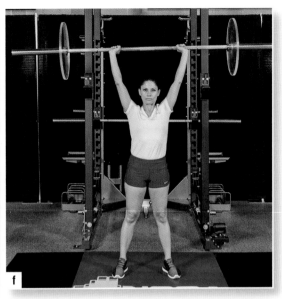

Figure 9.1 *(f)* Upper body pushing, vertically.

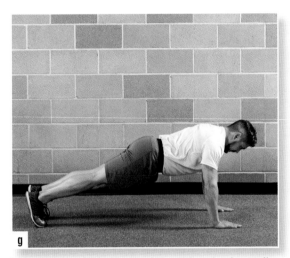

Figure 9.1 *(g)* Upper body pushing, horizontally.

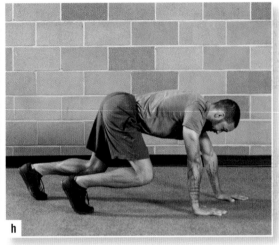

Figure 9.1 *(h)* Linear locomotion (crawling).

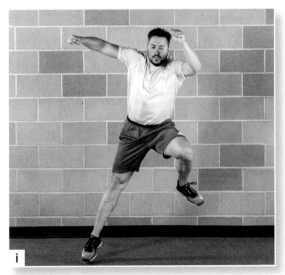

Figure 9.1 *(i)* Lateral locomotion.

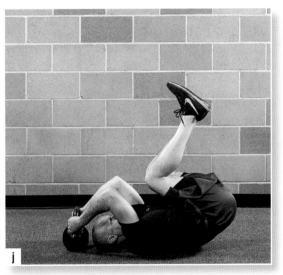

Figure 9.1 *(j)* Trunk flexion.

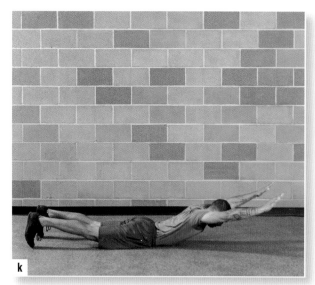

Figure 9.1 *(k)* Trunk extension.

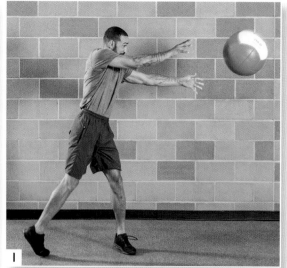

Figure 9.1 *(l)* Trunk rotation.

To achieve movement competency, you must first be able to achieve the positions involved in each movement. This requires adequate **flexibility**, mobility, and stability. Depending on who you ask, these qualities are subtlety different where *flexibility* involves the stretching of muscles while *mobility* refers to the range of motion about a joint. Regardless of differences in terminology, you need to be able to actively achieve proper end-range positions in a controlled, stable manner. Very few soldiering tasks are static (no movement); therefore, you need the ability to dynamically (with movement) transition between positions. This is referred to as **coordination** or **athleticism**. The ACFT tests athleticism.

MUSCULAR STRENGTH

Muscular strength is an expression of how much force can be applied to move an external object or one's own mass (for simplicity, *mass* is often referred to as *weight*). Force equals mass times acceleration ($F = m \times a$) where mass- is the object being moved and acceleration is typically represented by gravity. Strength is often discussed in absolute or relative terms. **Absolute strength** refers to the maximal force you can apply for one repetition, often referred to as your **one repetition maximum** (1RM). This is important for soldiers because when strength needs to be expressed on the battlefield, the object needing to be moved does not care how big or small you are (the enemy always gets a vote). Your ability to knock out 90 bodyweight push-ups in 2 minutes on the former APFT does not mean you possess the absolute strength needed to push a vehicle off a runway or help sustain movements under loads greater than 30 percent of your body weight. Similarly, many soldiers underappreciate absolute strength's contribution to endurance events. When each submaximal repetition occurs at a lower percentage of your 1RM, it causes less fatigue and makes the effort more sustainable.

Relative strength refers to how strong you are compared to your body weight. This is equally important as absolute strength because in many scenarios you need to maneuver your own mass over and around obstacles and arduous terrain. A 600-pound (273 kg) deadlift might not be worth chasing if that goal requires you to increase your body mass so much that you become insufficiently mobile in combat. However, superior maneuverability might become irrelevant if you do not possess the strength needed to extract a casualty.

Initially, absolute and relative strength can be increased simultaneously, but they may eventually compete with each other. Sometimes increasing absolute strength requires training hypertrophy to increase lean muscle mass. Contrarily, sometimes increasing relative strength requires training to reduce fat mass or, on very rare occasions, even decreasing lean mass. All mass comes at a metabolic cost, but a comprehensive conditioning program can effectively offset much of that cost. There is likely an ideal level of absolute strength and ratio of strength to mass for each MOS, but a good starting point is passing your job's minimum ACFT requirements for the MDL, SDC, and 2MR. Keep in mind that all ACFT events are influenced by strength, at least to some degree.

AEROBIC ENDURANCE

Aerobic endurance describes your ability to perform at a steady pace for a long duration and is essential for repetitive tasks like foot marching. The 2MR specifically tests aerobic endurance, and many Army schools still require completion of a five-mile run under a given time. Furthermore, aerobic endurance aids in recoverability between ACFT events, much like it helps lower the heart rate for improved execution of fine motor tasks after higher-intensity activities such as shooting accuracy after sprinting to cover. Typical PT programs in Army Basic Training aim to build conditioning by progressively increasing the distance of runs and ruck (foot) marches. This simple approach is likely very effective as long as runs and rucks are performed at the appropriate intensity for achievable distances. Increasing weekly volume by 10 percent or less is a good rule of thumb to prevent overtraining.

Both central (cardiorespiratory) and peripheral (skeletal muscle) factors contribute to your body's ability to deliver and utilize oxygen efficiently. This means that aerobic endurance training needs to address improving the performance of the heart and lungs and the specific muscles involved in the task for which you are training. Favorable adaptations of the heart increase its ability to deliver blood to the rest of the body. Low-intensity, long-duration steady-state training is the best way to improve this, while interval training can be a beneficial addition once simple progressions in distance and duration no longer yield observable progress. Common gauges to ensure the aerobic system is targeted during training include maintaining a certain percent of maximum heart rate (MHR) or simply keeping a pace at which you can comfortably have a conversation. A variety of modalities can be used to improve central aerobic contributors. However, adaptations are best trained by performing the specific task. For example, running improves running better than cycling because it has a higher level of specificity.

POWER

Power is an expression of force times velocity $(P = F \times v)$. Simply put, how much weight are you moving and how fast? Because power is comprised of both force and velocity, its maximization requires the application of both strength and speed qualities. Moving a lighter object at a high velocity biases the velocity portion of the equation, while moving a heavy object at a slower velocity biases the force portion. Increasing either force, velocity, or both without reducing the magnitude of its counterpart results in a higher power output. Strength and speed span a continuum from absolute strength, such as a 1RM deadlift, to absolute speed, such as in a golf swing (figure 9.2).

Strength-speed, closer to the high force output side of the continuum, is displayed by activities such as Olympic weightlifting. Contrarily, speed-strength, closer to the high velocity side of the continuum, is displayed by activities such as plyometrics (e.g., jumps, hops, bounds). Power output is maximized somewhere near the center of that continuum due to large contributions from both strength and speed.

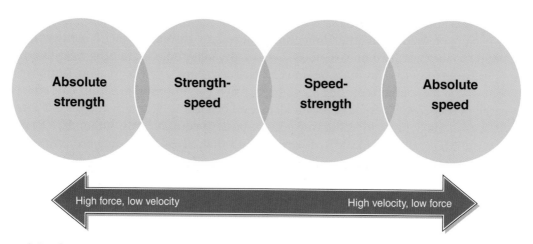

Figure 9.2   Strength and speed continuum.

Adapted by permission from National Strength and Conditioning Association, *Developing Power* (Champaign, IL: Human Kinetics, 2017), 191.

Likely due to the high volume of submaximal resistance moved at submaximal velocities in traditional APFT-focused PT, soldiers are commonly underpowered. Frankly, underpowered soldiers are either weak, slow, or both and the new ACFT is less forgiving of underpowered soldiers.

Training power typically involves multijoint exercises performed with a high rate of force development at various intensities for few repetitions with plenty of rest between sets.

SPEED AND AGILITY

Speed involves acceleration, maintenance of continuous (often top end) speed, and deceleration, all occurring in a linear fashion. *Speed* within this section refers to running speed. **Agility** often includes these same phases but executed multidirectionally. Technically, agility involves reacting to a stimulus and the term is used liberally here as a substitute for *change of direction*. The battlefield is three-dimensional, so testing speed and agility, primarily through the SDC, certainly relates to combat readiness. While it might be rare that a soldier needs to move at full speed, these performance components help prevent injury while traversing arduous terrain, particularly while loaded. Movement competency, strength, and power are all supportive components that are necessary to demonstrate proficiency in speed and agility. These supportive traits should be trained as a precursor to more specific drills. If you are strong and powerful and you move well, you are likely to achieve a decent score on the SDC, even if you do not specifically train speed and agility.

In the tactical setting, speed and agility are often trained with an emphasis on drills instead of skills; however, a large skill component requires shorter duration and fresh and focused execution with adequate rest between bouts to develop it effectively. Important underlying skills include the ability to accelerate and decelerate linearly, sprint at or near top speed, change direction, and move laterally. Ideally, these skills should be developed independently prior to adding complexity by combining them or performing them under fatigue. Some coaches make their living by fine-tuning their athletes' speed and agility because these components of performance are essential for success in so many sports. However, in the absence of in-person coaching, these skills can still be advanced effectively through simple exercises performed at maximum intensity.

ANAEROBIC ENDURANCE

Anaerobic endurance is a term that seems paradoxical because anaerobic bouts of performance are short in duration and high in intensity, while endurance implies a long duration bout at a submaximal intensity. *Anaerobic repeatability* might be a better phrase to describe your ability to maintain a high-intensity output over the course of repeated efforts with optimal or suboptimal rest between them. Several factors interact with one another to determine the quality of performance over subsequent anaerobic intervals.

The most influential factors are the intensity and duration of effort, the amount of rest between efforts, and your aerobic fitness. All of these factors contribute to your ability to buffer the byproducts that hinder your performance output. Higher intensities, longer (but still anaerobic) durations, short rest periods, and low aerobic capacity are factors that negatively affect how well you sustain quality of performance. Imagine sprinting one lap around a track as fast as possible, resting for only 30 seconds, and running another lap as fast as possible. The initial maximum-intensity, relatively long-duration effort with little rest before the subsequent sprint will make you unable to repeat that effort at the same speed for the second sprint. Contrarily, imagine sprinting only 5 yards (about 5 m) and then walking the remaining 95 yards (87 m) of the football field before turning around to do it again in the other direction. It is likely that you can repeat near the same quality of output for several intervals because even if the intensity is maximal, the duration is short and the rest is long.

One common misconception is that performing a set number of rounds for time or performing as many repetitions as possible (AMRAP) over a fixed duration qualifies as anaerobic endurance training. Performed with continuous effort, regardless of the exercises involved, these types of training sessions tend to occur below your body's anaerobic threshold, keeping them aerobic in nature. In reality, the anaerobic energy system can only contribute maximally to a few minutes of continuous high-intensity effort. Therefore, rest between exercise bouts is the key ingredient missing from an AMRAP or "for time" training session.

MUSCULAR ENDURANCE

Repeated movement of a submaximal load for a given number of repetitions or time, as well as an extended amount of time, is referred to as **muscular endurance**. The ACFT tests muscular endurance by requiring you to move your body weight for as many repetitions as possible during the HRP and LTK events. The HRP tests muscular endurance of your upper-body pushing muscles while the LTK tests muscular endurance of your trunk muscles, grip, and upper-body pulling muscles. Grip endurance is extremely important in many tactical activities but is often overlooked in training. As mentioned in chapter 6, findings by Major Donny Bigham, who tested more than 3,000 soldiers in four years, shows that a grip strength baseline of body weight and personal protective equipment (about 60 pounds [27 kg]) is needed by soldiers with highly physical jobs; however, less than 17 percent of soldiers tested achieve this.

Maintaining a lower body weight is advantageous for aerobic endurance activities. The SDC also involves muscular endurance of the lower body, but the event contains tasks in which a fixed load is moved in addition to body weight. Sometimes a higher body weight makes it easier to move external loads. Lean mass is preferred because it can be put to work compared to its more burdensome fat mass counterpart. Essentially, body composition can limit performance on muscular endurance–based events within the ACFT.

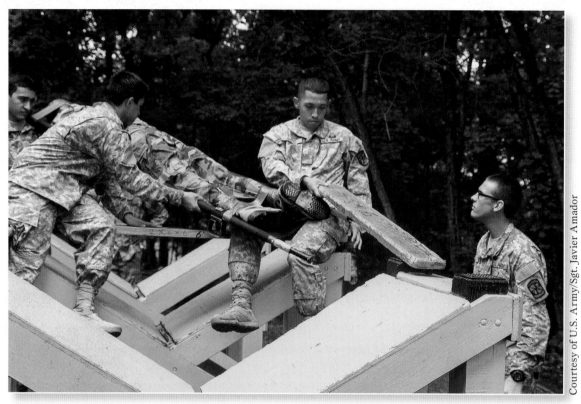

Courtesy of U.S. Army/Sgt. Javier Amador

Obstacle courses are often used to simulate combat conditions, and they require muscular endurance to traverse successfully.

Preparation and Programming

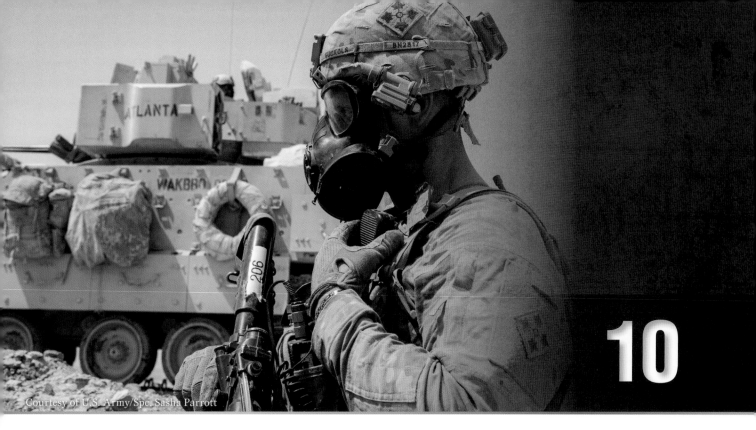

10

Your Current State of Readiness

The term **readiness** is often used within military dialogue and has been associated with more than one definition. Although the term is well suited for a variety of situations and circumstances, it is important to examine the true definition and determine an accurate definition as it relates to the ACFT.

DEFINING READINESS

The Oxford dictionary defines *readiness* as the "state of being fully prepared for something," whereas the Merriam-Webster dictionary defines it as "a quality or state of being ready: such as a state of preparation." Although very similar definitions, being fully prepared for something versus simply describing a state of preparation are entirely different. These differences in definition are also seen between the FM 7-22's definition of physical readiness and the ACFT scoring standards. FM 7-22, the Army's field manual governing PT, defines physical readiness as "the ability to meet the physical demands of any combat or duty position, accomplish the mission, and continue to fight and win." Contrarily, the ACFT scoring standards suggest levels of readiness based on minimum competency or performance levels for each event and overall performance, suggesting "prepared enough" instead of "fully prepared." It is difficult, if not impossible, to claim to be fully prepared in advance of any mission; therefore, the ACFT defines readiness as prepared enough or ill-prepared as it relates to the minimum standards set for each category based on MOS.

ASSESSMENT OF READINESS

The ACFT is a rather robust assessment because it assesses ten different components of physical fitness: power, muscular endurance, muscular strength, speed, agility, aerobic endurance, balance, flexibility, coordination, and reaction time. For the sake of simplicity, this text reduces those components to power, speed and agility, muscular strength, muscular endurance, anaerobic endurance, and aerobic endurance. Streamlining performance components allows the assessment results to be more easily understood and precisely related to prioritization of training needs.

The descriptions of *prepared* or *ill-prepared* now shift to a focus of pursuing maintenance or enhancement. Maintaining readiness suggests that your current state is at or above the minimum standard for all the events and you do not desire to improve your scores. Enhancing readiness is your focus when looking to improve your score, regardless of how it compares to the standards. It is crucial that you perform an assessment to determine the direction and priorities of your training.

The purpose of an assessment such as the ACFT is to reduce the number of events to the fewest necessary to evaluate required performance components; it is not to encourage the assessment exercise as the sole means of training. Therefore, it is important to understand the primary fitness components being assessed by each event (table 10.1) and focus on improving or maintaining each of them, not just the assessed exercise. For example, use exercises such as lunges, squats, or Romanian deadlifts to improve lower-body strength associated with the MDL, rather than simply training the MDL by itself. The inclusion of variety in training to develop lower-body strength, and consequently the MDL, also provides movement variability that translates even better to combat scenarios than the MDL alone. In fact, even the best deadlifters in the world use complementary and accessory exercises to improve their world-record deadlifts. This further suggests the need for variety within your physical training plan, even when an exercise in itself is the only driver of training.

The need for variety and movement variability holds true for each of the ACFT events' tested components of performance. The ACFT is reduced to the fewest number of exercises needed to assess the underlying performance components that you need as a soldier; it is not meant to serve as the training means for complete physical development.

Table 10.1   Fitness Components by Event

Fitness component	ACFT event
Muscular endurance	Hand Release Push-Up–Arm Extension, Leg Tuck*
Muscular strength	3 Repetition Maximum Deadlift, Leg Tuck*
Power	Standing Power Throw
Anaerobic endurance	Sprint-Drag-Carry
Aerobic endurance	Two-Mile Run

*When the number of LTK repetitions performed is low or even unachievable, the test becomes an additional assessment of muscular strength rather than muscular endurance.

EVALUATING AND INTERPRETING RESULTS

After performing the assessment, you must evaluate and interpret your results to appropriately prioritize needs and guide the structure of your PT. Evaluating results refers to relating the score for each event to the standards associated with your MOS' specific category, and ranking scores in order of lowest to highest. Interpreting results refers to taking a deeper look and considering how the components of performance assessed by each event relate to one another.

Evaluating your ACFT scores is as simple as looking at them at the surface level. If you score below your MOS' standard for any event, that or those events will obviously need to be a focus within your program. Rank each event based on score alone, ordering them from lowest to highest. This will order the events and, as a result, their underlying performance components, which will help you determine how to prioritize them in your training plan. This simple evaluation process holds true if you score below the standard on one or multiple events. It also holds true if you score above the standard on all events and are pursuing a more physically well-rounded version of yourself. If you score well above the standard on all events, you can prioritize based on preference.

Interpreting the results requires a deeper understanding of how the primary components of performance for each event relate to one another and whether they are mutually beneficial. We will dive into the how the primary components of performance assessed during the ACFT relate to each other.

The components of performance were detailed in chapter 9 and are summarized here. Muscular strength is the ability to produce force. Muscular endurance is essentially the ability to produce force repeatedly. Power is an expression of force times velocity. Anaerobic endurance in function and in definition can be expanded upon, but regarding the ACFT it is the ability to produce a specific amount of work in the shortest amount of time possible. Aerobic endurance describes the ability to perform long duration activities at a steady pace, and also supports your ability to recover between events. These brief summaries begin to interrelate the components of performance.

Let's examine how they relate to the specific events so that you can interpret your results in a way that allows the best direction possible.

The MDL is an obvious assessment of muscular strength. If the performance on this event is a training priority based on your evaluation, you need to prioritize muscular strength. None of the other components of performance directly assessed by the ACFT drive this event's success. (Understand that movement competency, although not directly assessed by the ACFT, can relate to the MDL. If you are restricted or cannot get into the proper position with ease, this component should find its place in your training). However, muscular strength relates to components of performance assessed by several of the ACFT events that follow the MDL.

The SPT is an assessment of power. Power is one of the primary components of performance assessed by the ACFT and should be a focus of training if scores are below standard or if it is a high priority based on your initial evaluation. Training for this component specifically will be targeted through jumps, throws, and other explosive exercises that work to enhance the rate of force production. This is where a key perspective comes into play when interpreting your results. The ability to produce force (muscular strength) precedes the ability to produce force rapidly. So if the SPT and MDL are events you need to improve, you will be targeting both improvements through muscular strength–focused training. If your MDL score heavily outweighs your SPT score, then the previously mentioned jumps, throws, and other explosive exercises will be your priority for improving this component.

The HRP is an assessment of muscular endurance. Muscular endurance is also a primary component of performance assessed by the ACFT and is assessed by multiple events. If this component ranks high in your training priorities, it will best be targeted by submaximal

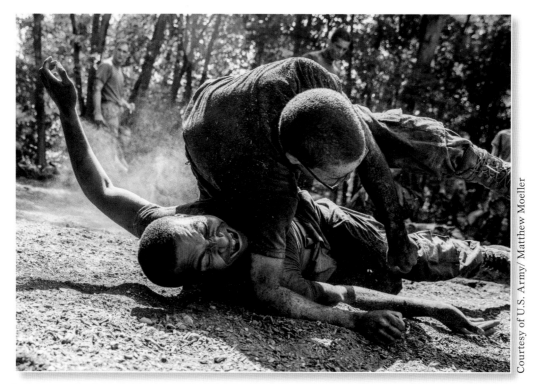

Courtesy of U.S. Army/ Matthew Moeller

Combatives require the expression of total body power to execute effective takedowns and strikes.

efforts typically repeated at or near your desired performance on the test. There are two additional factors that come into play when looking to improve this component as it relates to this event: muscular strength and body composition. **Body composition** describes what the body is made of that, at its most simple definition, is divided into two components: fat mass and fat-free mass. Generally speaking, the more muscular strength you have relative to your body weight, the more repetitions you will be able to perform in this event. If both the MDL and HRP are events that you need to prioritize, this highlights the need to focus first on muscular strength and then on muscular endurance. If your MDL score is good but your HRP score needs to be improved, changing your body composition (to reduce fat mass, increase fat-free mass—such as muscle—or both) should improve that score. Often, upper-body muscular strength (specifically horizontal pushing) is the limiting factor and should be focused on.

The LTK is also intended as an assessment of muscular endurance. But some soldiers cannot complete enough repetitions to demonstrate muscular endurance, so the LTK becomes an assessment of muscular strength instead. Even passing scores of 1, 3, and 5 repetitions, earning scores of 60, 65, and 70 points respectively, are not high enough to require true muscular endurance. A maximum score of 20 repetitions is an example of muscular endurance, however. The relationship between muscular strength and muscular endurance, as outlined for the HRP, still holds true in this scenario. There are also times in this scenario when the repetitions performed are low enough or even unachievable, which makes it an additional assessment of muscular strength rather than muscular endurance. If your MDL does not need to be a priority based on your initial evaluation but the LTK does, it is important to examine the likelihood of a body composition limitation. If this does not fit your specific situation, upper-body muscular strength (specifically vertical pulling) is likely the limiter and should be targeted accordingly.

The SDC is intended to assess multiple primary fitness components. This also makes it difficult to pinpoint the specific component needed to influence performance in this event without first interpreting the scores across all the events. Muscular strength will be more accurately assessed during the MDL. Muscular endurance is assessed in previous events although with an upper-body bias, pointing out the performance limiters that likely influence performance in this event as well. So if the events that assess muscular strength and muscular endurance need to be prioritized, it is likely this event will need some work too. If events that assess those two components outscore the SDC, it is likely anaerobic endurance—the component unique to this event—that is the limiter. If this is the case, training to enhance this will take place through efforts carried out at maximal or near-maximal effort for 30 seconds to 3 minutes in similar or relatable activities.

The 2MR is an assessment of aerobic endurance. There are several ways to assess aerobic endurance and an equal or greater number of ways it factors into performance scenarios. For the ACFT, aerobic endurance is directly assessed in real time through the sustainable pace maintained during the 2MR or the overall time. It is also being assessed indirectly throughout the ACFT because it is the component that facilitates recovery between each of the events. The less aerobic endurance you have, the less you will be able to display your true maximum effort for each subsequent event. If your 2MR suggests a need to prioritize aerobic endurance in your training, it is important to relate the time achieved during that run compared to a similar run performed in a standalone scenario. If the two are relatively close to each other, you need to focus on aerobic endurance with a bias toward running. If your standalone time is substantially better than your 2MR during the ACFT (for example, faster by more than a minute), you might need to focus your aerobic endurance efforts toward what is often referred to as work capacity. In this regard, work capacity refers to designing your training in a fashion that relates to the ACFT in its entirety. You will best be served by designing a program with daily sessions that are 60 to 75 minutes long (90 minutes if you want to stick to Army rules) and include a variety of movements and contractions that allow fatigue to accumulate in a similar fashion to the ACFT. Aerobic endurance from running alone will not solve the need for this component as it relates to work capacity.

Although body composition is not a component of performance outlined in this book, nor is it directly assessed by the events included in the ACFT, it plays a big role in your success and longevity. The influence of body composition has already been discussed in the HRP and LTK, and it also plays a role during the SDC to some degree. However, its influence on aerobic endurance shown in the 2MR is substantial. Often the fastest and most effective way to improve your 2MR is by adjusting your diet when body composition is a concern.

RETESTING

As of the date of publication, current AR 350-15 authorizes a minimum of 7 days and maximum of 24 days after the initial failure. It is unknown whether the Army will sustain this current policy, but a rewrite of *FM 7-22: Physical Readiness Training* around February 2020 should clarify. The ACFT will not affect soldiers' potential or careers until October 2021, which means they will have to pass the ACFT two times in that calendar year.

Failing the ACFT initiates the process of retesting. If failed, the ACFT must be retaken in its entirety within a certain time frame of the failed test. The US Army ACFT Field Testing Manual (2018) emphasizes that minimum rest periods between events need to be adhered to during retesting and that retests are "individually administered and scored." Scores on retests will undoubtedly undergo a higher level of scrutiny than initial scores because passing and failing have the potential to affect your career and promotion status.

Failing the ACFT also initiates the need to create and enact an effective training plan to improve the chance of passing the retest. Fortunately, chapter 12 contains specific plans that account for a variety of timelines and training frequencies to meet your needs. The current chapter already discussed how to evaluate and interpret results to prioritize the focus of training. Even if you are unable to follow prescribed training plans in their entirety, you can bias the components of performance that address your ACFT shortcomings. For example, if you performed well on events that emphasize muscular strength, it makes more sense to choose a conditioning-focused day instead of playing to your strengths and prioritizing resistance training. If you failed all the events, muscular strength and aerobic endurance possess the greatest carryover to all events. It is rare that a soldier with a solid foundation of both of these qualities does not also perform well on events that require muscular and anaerobic endurance and power.

While this book is a sound resource for ACFT training, qualified and certified coaching is irreplaceable. If you are struggling with where to begin in the remedial physical training process, seek out a professional strength and conditioning coach (preferably with military coaching experience) to help guide you in the right direction. Contact the Tactical Program at the National Strength and Conditioning Association (NSCA) for more information regarding additional coaching resources to better individualize your training. If you prefer to train on your own, the Volt Athletics training app provides the programming from this book within an app for your mobile device (see page 284).

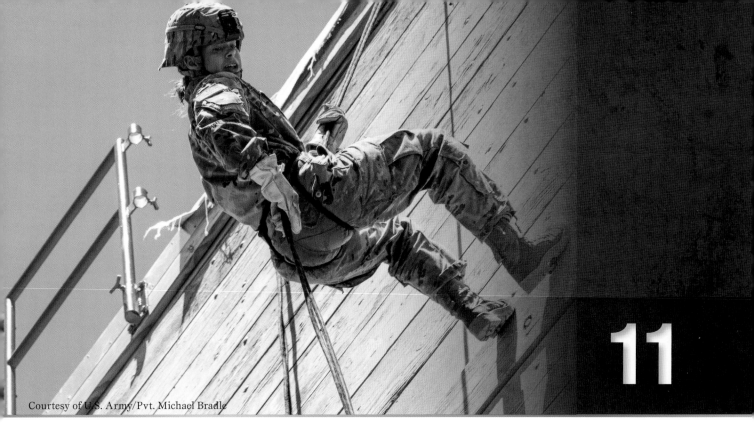

11

Training Plan Considerations

SAFETY RECOMMENDATIONS

Your safety should never be compromised for the sake of PT. The point of following a professionally designed program is to achieve performance gains in a predictably safe and effective manner that progressively overloads the body in accordance with evidence-based principles of strength and conditioning. Some general safety guidelines facilitate success, particularly when training in a group setting:

1. Train under the supervision of a certified professional when available.
2. Do not train through pain.
3. Select exercises, volumes, and intensities that allow for proper positions and execution.
4. Ensure adequate space for each soldier performing exercises, specifically

   - 3 feet (1 m) between ends of barbells and dumbbells,
   - 4 feet (about 1 m) around weightlifting platforms, and
   - 49 square feet (4.6 sq m) (7 ft × 7 ft [2 m × 2 m]) per solider for warm-up, cool-down, and calisthenics.

5. Use equipment from reputable companies for its intended purpose only and inspect it regularly.

TIME UNTIL TEST DATE

This book contains a number of training plans in chapter 12 based on the time remaining until your test date. More time allowed reduces the risk of injury by providing the luxury of gradual progression in training volume and intensity. When testing with extremely short notice, you should prioritize familiarizing yourself with each test event. Familiarity with and practice of each event can reduce your test anxiety and even add a few points to your score when there is not sufficient time to truly improve your physical abilities. When a little more lead time is available, focusing on the performance components of total-body muscular strength and aerobic endurance (specifically running) will generally have positive carryover to the greatest number of events. However, the ACFT is not a test for which you want to procrastinate your preparation. Plan ahead and use as much time as possible to train intelligently.

INDIVIDUAL CONSIDERATIONS

Each person will have a unique set of circumstances that affect the training program. This section describes them one at a time; be sure to consider all of these factors before you start training and refer to them as needed as you progress through your program.

Competing Demands

While the time remaining until your test date might be the primary driver behind the length of your selected training plan, competing demands dictate how frequently you train due to their demand on your time and ability to recover. A long road march does not lend itself favorably to a lower-body strength training session the following day, just like a long night at the range does not set you up for maximal-intensity speed and agility training the next morning. The number of days assigned in sessions within this book does not come with consideration for competing demands. You will need to recognize them and make the necessary adjustments to ensure your training is safe, effective, and allows for the recovery needed to realize positive adaptations.

Sometimes competing demands provide a substitute or an additional training session. If you have an unavoidable company-level five-mile run on a Friday morning, it can serve as an aerobic endurance session. Perhaps this session replaces an existing one in your program if you do not have the time to complete both or cannot add an extra day to develop this essential component of performance. Some competing demands simply compete for your time and have no physical benefit. In these cases, follow the guidance provided in chapter 10 and prioritize the days of the plan that best target your weakest performance attributes. If you are a good distance runner and find yourself pressed for time, your tendency will be to default to going for a run; however, you need to resist this temptation in favor of a resistance training session that develops your strength and power shortcomings.

Fitness Level

Your current fitness level influences the frequency, intensity, and volume of your training. If you currently possess a low level of fitness, it might be best to resist training five days per week, even if your schedule allows for it. If you do train with high frequency, consider keeping one or two of those sessions lighter in intensity or lower in volume to reduce risk of injury. Your intensity in terms of speed and load is fairly self-regulating and will be lower than a fitter version of yourself; however, if you used to possess a higher level of fitness, resist the temptation to try to match your previous intensities. Volume is another variable to adjust based on fitness level. The training plans within this book progress volume as systematically as possible based on the length of program. Increasing volume slowly over a longer time period is safer and more sustainable than jumping into higher training volumes too quickly. Trying to do too much too soon is a primary precursor to both acute and chronic injuries that can reduce or completely curb the effectiveness of your training.

Training Age or IQ

While fitness level influences your capacity for training, your training age and training IQ determine how skillfully you execute the exercises within your program. More experienced individuals with higher training IQ's perform exercises more efficiently than novices. Soldiers with extensive or high-level athletic backgrounds likely perform speed and agility drills more efficiently than soldiers without much experience in multidirectional sports. Note that your training age is specific to the type of training with which you have experience. Your history as an elite cross-country runner, for example, does not necessarily translate to proficiency in strength training any more than a history in powerlifting translates to a rhythmic display of agility. Some soldiers possess high levels of natural strength and power but have an inability to harness it effectively because they are new to skills involved in training. Meanwhile, an experienced weightlifter with a high training IQ could take years off from training and still possess the muscle memory to perform the exercises with a decent level of proficiency.

Available Training Time

The Army has a tendency to place excessive time demands on its soldiers that reduce your availability for PT. Two primary time considerations are **frequency** and **duration** (how often and for how long). The training sessions in this book are already adjusted and prioritized for as many as five and as few as two days per week and fit easily within a typical PT session. However, you might have weeks when you have fewer days to train than expected, a shorter duration in which to fit a session, or both. No perfect solution exists for these scenarios, but the simple alternative is to prioritize the training sessions or pieces of your sessions that address your weaknesses. Resist the temptation to fall back on the type of training with which you are most comfortable and familiar. It takes much less time and effort to maintain your strengths than it does to develop your weaknesses. Keep in mind that consistency is paramount for positive change in training. Three 30-minute sessions within a week are more effective than one 90-minute session.

Environment, Seasonality, and Location

Environmental considerations and constraints will influence your training plan. Extremely hot environments might require your conditioning to be performed while it is dark outside or in an air-conditioned indoor setting. Also, extreme cold or snow might prevent outdoor training altogether and force you to compete for time in crowded Morale, Welfare, and Recreation (MWR) gyms. Look for opportunities instead of excuses, but do not place yourself or your soldiers in precarious environmental conditions. Environmental extremes like hot, cold, and altitude require purposeful and progressive acclimation. Follow Army doctrine for proper acclimation and hydration protocols for various environments.

Access to Equipment

Equipment availability is one of, if not the most frequently, referenced issues facing soldiers looking to train effectively for the ACFT. The Army is slowly working to address this problem, but in the meantime some creativity might be necessary to overcome it. The exercises within this book purposely require simple equipment such as barbells and dumbbells; however, while this equipment is common in athletic settings, typical military gyms often come up short because these items were not necessary for training to pass the APFT in the past. In recognition of equipment shortcomings, the exercises within this book can easily be substituted. When the prescribed equipment is not available, reference the exercise section with the same movement as the prescribed exercise and select an alternative based on what you do have available. Included within each movement type, you will find exercises that cover a majority of common equipment options and include body weight when absolutely no equipment is available.

Injury and Health Status

Do not perform exercises that are contraindicated based on your injury or health status. However, do not use an ailment you can train around safely as a crutch when training alternatives are available. If you are injured, follow the proper channels to see your unit's physical therapist or athletic trainer to help determine what components of your training are still safe to perform. If you are sick, follow your unit's medical protocol to receive an appropriate and effective level of care. It almost never pays off to train through pain or illness, nor is it often necessary.

RECOVERY

Positive adaptations to the stress applied during training do not occur during training itself. Instead, they happen during between training sessions when your body is able to recover. The ACFT preparation program within this book does not prescribe specific recovery sessions, but preventing the negative physical effects associated with overtraining requires implementing recovery methods. The goal of recovery is to maximize positive training effects by mitigating fatigue induced by chronic training. Following a progressive and periodized training plan like the one within this book reduces the risk of overtraining. Weeks that *deload*, or reduce volume or intensity (or both) of training, allow your body to recover from the overload applied in weeks prior to the deload week. However, some other recovery options are worth mentioning.

Nutrition

This book is not a manual for ideal dietary intake. Please see the Suggested Resources section in this book for books that specifically address nutrition. That said, it is essential that you hydrate and fuel your body appropriately to facilitate recovery and achieve supercompensation. Quantity and quality of your caloric intake helps your body build back up from the breakdown experienced during training. This rebuilding process is essential for maximizing strength and endurance by optimizing body composition and energy levels. The proper amount and ratios of carbohydrate, fat, and protein are vital to realizing training benefits. Most units have a registered dietitian you can consult for specific guidance.

Sleep

The ability to achieve a sound and sufficient night's sleep often eludes soldiers because of late nights, early mornings, professional and personal stress, poor nutrition, and irregular schedules. Much like nutrition, you need to strive to enhance your sleep quantity and quality to properly recover and optimize your performance. Adequate sleep is necessary for physical and cognitive function, with negative effects of sleep deprivation having strong similarities to impairment caused by drinking alcohol. The American Sleep Association recommends 7 to 8 hours of sleep per night for most adults, but some need as high as 10. Sleep quality can be enhanced by practicing good sleep hygiene, which simply means having a pre-bed routine that leads to better sleep. Things to refrain from include late-night screen time and eating, caffeinated beverages after noon, alcohol, and tobacco products. Practices to promote improved sleep quality include a dark, quiet, and cool room; regular exercise (preferably not too close to bedtime); and other means of mitigating stress, such as meditation. If you think you have sleep issues, seek professional analysis and guidance, which are often free for soldiers on most installations.

Active Recovery Sessions

Many recovery modalities and devices are popularized due to social media, some of which are quite expensive. However, inexpensive options exist and can be extremely beneficial in aiding in recovery. Common commercialized options include various forms or cryo-, hydro-, and thermotherapy; massage; and compression garments. You are welcome to learn about the efficacy of these recovery interventions and incorporate them into your training as desired. Some of the suggested resources suggested within this book contain research-based insight into their effectiveness.

The suggestion of this book is to simply incorporate standalone sessions into your training that emphasize movement quality, through a full range of motion, and in a deloaded state. In other words, take yourself from start to finish through a thorough warm-up, possibly preceded by some full-body foam rolling that specifically targets any muscles that feel abnormally tight. Similarly, an instructor-led yoga session might be beneficial. Recovery through the practice of diaphragmatic breathing techniques can help your body shift from a stressed sympathetic state to a more relaxed parasympathetic state. Another suggestion for deloading the body is to get off your feet and incorporate the occasional pool session as a means of low-intensity aerobic endurance training. If you do not know how to swim well, simply perform the upright portions of the warm-up routine found within this book in the shallow end of the pool.

Keep in mind the ultimate goal of recovery is to reduce the negative effects of training stress on your body and not to create new stress that requires additional recovery time and energy. Reducing or removing physical stressors through planned deload periods and true days off is paramount. Nurturing your body with appropriate quantity and quality of food and sleep are great passive forms of recovery. Purposeful, unloaded active recovery methods like massage, movement sessions, and breathing or meditation can be injected almost anywhere into your training routine.

POST–ARMY COMBAT FITNESS TEST MAINTENANCE

The goal of this book is to prepare you specifically to perform your best on the ACFT. While training for the test and training for your job are not nearly as divided as they were when the former APFT was the testing standard, this program might not address some considerations regarding task specificity. In the absence of qualified professional guidance, repeating the program in this book after applying your newfound physicality to the ACFT could continue to advance your physical performance levels. While the set and repetition guidelines remain unchanged, the intensities of your resistance training exercises and your conditioning efforts will be executed as a percentage of a higher maximum, thereby facilitating continued progress. More certainly, if you become deconditioned after a period of insufficient or inconsistent training, repeating one of the sample programs in this book is an appropriate way to regain your physical ability levels. The more advanced you are, the more individualized training you will need to continue to progress. Look to the Suggested Resources section at the end of this book for more advanced training options or additional avenues for further training.

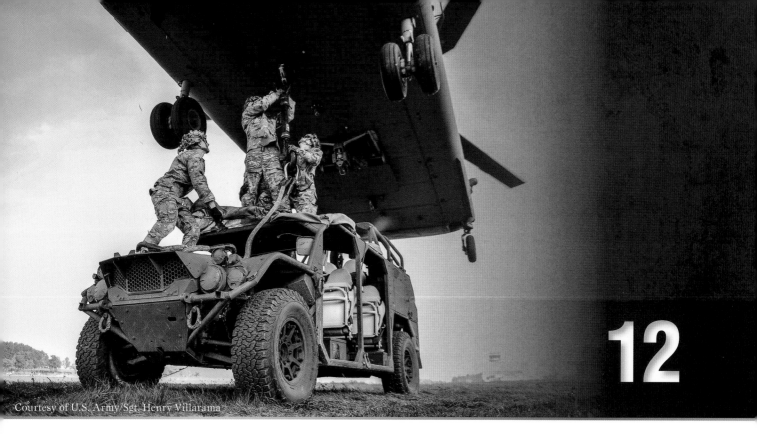

Courtesy of U.S. Army/Sgt. Henry Villarama

Sample Training Plans

The training programs within this chapter offer enough flexibility that lack of time or equipment is no excuse for failing the ACFT. Each 24-week, 12-week, 8-week, and 4-week plan in this chapter offers a 5-, 4-, 3-, and 2-days-per-week option. Cramming is not a reliable way to study for a test, nor is it the ideal way to approach training for the ACFT. A crash course of eight weeks or less might suffice if you are already physically fit and simply need to better understand how to execute the ACFT's events. However, training for the full 24 weeks at a rate of only 2 days per week is more beneficial than a 4-week program of 5 days per week. Slow progress is sustainable progress, and you are less likely to sustain an injury during training when you allow time for proper progression.

We will discuss the steps for selecting which program to execute and how to adjust when life gets in the way. Afterward, we will address how to execute the exercises within the program and the best approach to substituting what is prescribed when assigned equipment is inaccessible.

SELECTING AND ADJUSTING A TRAINING PLAN

1. **Select the program with the training frequency of days per week you can most likely accomplish.**

   Do not choose the five-days-per-week option just because you want to train five days per week. Pick the frequency that best suits your reality in terms of schedule and competing demands. The lower frequency training options keep essential components while reducing less vital exercises, so a three-days-per-week program can still greatly improve your performance over the course of your training. The program does not assign specific days of the week to train because it needs to remain flexible to adapt to the common inconsistency of Army scheduling. Ideally, you would space your training days out to maximize recovery; however, get in your training when you can even if ideal is not a possibility. For example, if you can only train two days per week, a Monday-Thursday split would maximize recovery, but if, in a given week, only Monday and Tuesday are available, training on back-to-back days trumps only training one day that week.

2. **Choose the longest training duration possible leading up to your ACFT.**

   If you are doing the full 24-week program, you will simply follow the program from phase 1, day 1 through the final day of phase 6. If you are doing a 12-, 8-, or 4-week program due to time constraints, use table 12.1 to determine the order of phases and weeks within those phases. They are all derived from the original 24-week program.

Table 12.1   12-, 8-, and 4-Week Versions of the 24-Week Training Program

Number of weeks to the ACFT date*	12-week training program	8-week training program	4-week training program
12	P1 W1		
11	P1 W2		
10	P1 W3		
9	P2 W1		
8	P2 W3	P1 W1	
7	P2 W4	P1 W2	
6	P5 W2	P5 W1	
5	P5 W3	P5 W2	
4	P5 W4	P5 W3	P6 W1
3	P6 W1	P1 W1	P6 W2
2	P6 W2	P6 W2	P6 W3
1	P6 W4	P6 W4	P6 W4

If you are doing the full 24-week program, follow the program from phase 1, day 1 through the final day of phase 6. Only use this table for a 12-, 8-, or 4-week version of the full 24-week program.

P = phase

W = week

3. **Adjust the frequency of your training as scheduling issues present themselves.**
Regardless of which frequency you choose upfront, you can always adjust on a week-to-week basis as needed. In other words, if you regularly train with a four-days-per-week program but know that you will only be able to accomplish two days in an upcoming week, it is likely best that you complete the same phase and week of training but with the two-day option instead of the four. Those two days will likely contain more of what you need than randomly selecting two days from your four-day option. That said, if you do need to pick two days from a higher frequency program, pick at least one that addresses your greatest weakness. Both maximum strength and aerobic endurance have decent shelf lives, so they can be sidelined for a week or two due to disrupted training while you spend your limited training opportunities on your weaker of the two.

EXERCISE EXECUTION

Prior to each training session, follow the warm-up guidance within chapter 13. It will ensure you are prepared to maximize the potential of your session. Typically, whether your session is solely strength, solely conditioning, or a combination of the two, your warm-up will segue immediately into some sort of power movement such as a jump, throw, or weightlifting variation. These exercises should be executed with the intent to develop force rapidly. The goal of the strength-focused exercises afterward is force production, so you want to achieve as heavy a load as possible for the repetitions assigned, without uncertainty as to whether you will complete all the assigned repetitions. For all exercises within your selected program, proper technique is paramount. Do not let your need to produce speed or strength compromise the quality of exercise execution. Some days are conditioning focused, while others finish with a shorter bout of conditioning work.

Keep in mind that not every single session is meant to be performed at maximum intensity. Follow lifting intensity guidelines where provided within the program, and, especially when performing a high number of sessions in a week (four to five), only perform one of them at an absolute all-out effort. However, most sessions should still require just shy of maximal effort, and you might leave 1 to 2 repetitions still in the tank each set. For conditioning exercises, follow the prescription given because it is purposely polarized, with some days being extremely uncomfortable and others being easier than you are used to.

For the resistance training exercises, here are some things to note:

■ **Italicized versus nonitalicized sets × repetitions.** When an exercise has both italicized and nonitalicized sets × repetitions listed next to it, the italicized sets are *warm-up sets*, and the nonitalicized sets are *working (training) sets*. When there are only nonitalicized sets listed, they are all working sets.

■ **Percent of an ACFT event.** Sometimes when the push-up or deadlift exercise is listed in a program, the assigned intensity is based on a percent of an ACFT event such as the number of HRP repetitions (for the push-up) or the MDL weight (for the deadlift). Ideally, you would have taken the ACFT recently so your HRP and MDL scores reflect your current fitness level for those events. If you have never taken the ACFT, go back to chapter 10 to determine your current state of readiness.

■ **Work up to an RM.** When the program requests that you work up to a 1, 3, or 5RM (i.e., a *repetition maximum*, meaning the most weight you can lift for 1, 3, or 5 repetitions), you will take several sets to do so. These sets should be preceded by the warm-up set or sets listed with the first attempt to determine your maximum for the number of repetitions listed being a *conservative* first RM attempt. If the conservative attempt is easy, add weight and perform a more aggressive second attempt. Allow at least a two-minute rest between attempts and do not perform more than three RM attempts. Exercises that include a work up to an RM often include additional subsequent sets using a weight that is at a certain percentage of the RM. Simply multiply the RM load you achieved by the assigned percentage to determine the weight to use in the subsequent sets.

■ **Supersets**. You will often perform two to three exercises in a paired or small circuit fashion. These supersets will be depicted by the number preceding the exercises. For example, "2a" and "2b" should be performed in an alternating fashion, while "3a, 3b, 3c" should be performed in a circuit fashion. Some exercises will not be supersetted, but many, if not most, will be.

■ **Rest**. Unless otherwise stated, rest enough between exercises to allow for a strong effort on all repetitions. This is especially important for the heavier exercises that fall immediately after the power exercises. As the workout transitions from heavier compound exercises that use multiple joints and muscle groups to accessory exercises that are less taxing on the system, you can reduce your rest between sets and exercises.

■ **Deload weeks**. The fourth week of most phases is a *deload week*, when volume is reduced compared to the preceding weeks. Resist the urge to do more sets and repetitions than the program prescribes because the deload purposefully helps your body recover from the progressive overload applied during previous weeks. You still want to maintain fairly high intensity this week, but it is OK if you want to take a little bit of the edge off with a slight intensity reduction.

■ **Abbreviated sessions**. Ideally, you will execute each day in its entirety throughout the program; however, sometimes time does not allow for completing every exercise, set, and repetition. In these cases, try to complete the power exercises and the heavier strength exercises. After those are complete, you need to decide whether to prioritize the accessory exercises or conditioning. Look to chapter 10 for what to dedicate your remaining time to. Typically, you will address your weakness first. If you scored poorly on conditioning events, you should prioritize conditioning, but if you scored poorly on strength-based events, you should prioritize the accessory resistance training instead. Keep in mind that maintaining current strengths takes a smaller dose than trying to move the needle positively on your weaknesses.

PROGRAM ACRONYMS

The program is full of acronyms to help guide exercise equipment selection and execution.

EQUIPMENT

BB: barbell

DB: dumbbell

KB: kettlebell

MB: medicine ball

SB: stability ball

EXECUTION

Alt (alternating): Alternate repetitions between one side and the other side of the body.

AMRAP (as many repetitions as possible): Perform as many repetitions as you possibly can for that set.

ECC (eccentric emphasis): Move intentionally slowly when moving the same direction that the resistance is trying to move you (typically down with gravity). ECC will typically be followed by a number that represents the number of seconds to control the movement eccentrically. For example, "ECC3" means to control the eccentric portion of the lift for three seconds.

EMOM (every minute on the minute): Perform the corresponding circuit or exercise at the top of each minute for the prescribed number of total minutes.

ISO (isometric): Hold in the transitional position for the number of seconds prescribed. For example, "ISO3" means to hold the transitional portion of the exercise for three seconds. The transitional position is either between the eccentric movement and the concentric movement, such as the bottom of a push-up, or between the concentric movement and the eccentric movement, such as the top of a pull-up. It is the transitional position that requires the most work to fight against gravity and is typically the bottom portion of an exercise.

SA (single arm): Perform the exercise on one side before transitioning and performing the exercise on the opposite side arm.

SL (single leg): Perform the exercise on one side before transitioning and performing the exercise on the opposite side leg.

MR (multiple response): Perform the repetitions continuously without a pause in the landing position.

RDL: Romanian deadllift

RFE: rear foot elevated

RG (reverse grip): Perform the exercise with a supinated (palms-up) grip.

SR (single response): Perform the repetitions one at a time with a pause in the landing position.

Wtd: weighted

Exercise Finder

The resistance training exercises and conditioning drills in this list were assembled from the sample programs and often they are specific versions of the more general exercises and drills described in the chapters in part IV.

EXERCISE SUBSTITUTIONS AND CHOOSING ALTERNATIVE EXERCISES

The exercises included in the chapter 12 programs are the preferred exercises as they relate to the ACFT and the program as a whole. If an alternative exercise is needed (due to equipment or space limitations, for example), you will need to select an alternative exercise from an exercise chapter. Go to the table at the start of the chapter that includes the preferred exercise and find the exercise you need to replace along the top row. (The name will not include the piece of equipment being used.) Next, find the equipment options to which you have access along the left-hand column. Your exercise alternative options are the cells where the exercise you are replacing and the types of equipment to which you have access intersect on the table. Choose the option that best mimics the position, movement, and resistance level of the assigned exercise. Note that not every type of equipment supports an alternative, but at least one body weight replacement exists for every exercise, so there is no excuse to omit a programmed exercise entirely. Once you have selected a replacement exercise, you can reference detailed instructions on how to perform it within the exercise chapters.

Table 12.2   Two-Day Program, Phase 1

WEEK 1			
Day 1		**Day 2**	
(1) Vertical jump	2 × 5 (SR)	(1) Vertical jump	2 × 5 (SR)
(2a) DB walking lunge	*1 × 8 each* 3 × 12 each	(2a) Deadlift	2 × 5
(2b) Shoulder press	*2 × 5* 3 × 10	(2b) Push-up	2 × 10
(2c) Ab rollout	3 × 12	**(3) EMOM circuit:**	15 min
(3a) Pull-up	*2 × 5* 3 × 10	(a) Deadlift	× 2 @ 74% of ACFT MDL weight
(3b) SB leg curl	3 × 12	(b) Push-up	15% of ACFT HRP reps
(3c) Front plank	3 × 30 sec	(4a) Inverted row	3 × 12
		(4b) Reverse crunch	3 × 12
		(5a) Facepull	3 × 12
		(5b) Side bend	3 × 12 each
Conditioning		**Conditioning**	
100 yd shuttle (in 25 yd increments)	× 6 with 2:30 rest	3-5 mile run	70%-80% MHR
WEEK 2			
Day 1		**Day 2**	
(1) Vertical jump	2 × 5 (SR)	(1) Vertical jump	2 × 5 (SR)
(2a) DB walking lunge	*1 × 8 each* 3 × 12 each	(2a) Deadlift	2 × 5
(2b) Shoulder press	*2 × 5* 3 × 10	(2b) Push-up	2 × 10
(2c) Ab rollout	3 × 12	**(3) EMOM circuit:**	20 min
(3a) Pull-up	*2 × 5* 3 × 10	(a) Deadlift	× 2 @ 74% of ACFT MDL weight
(3b) SB leg curl	3 × 12	(b) Push-up	15% of ACFT HRP reps
(3c) Front plank	3 × 30 sec	(4a) Inverted row	3 × 12
		(4b) Reverse crunch	3 × 12
		(5a) Facepull	3 × 12
		(5b) Side bend	3 × 12 each
Conditioning		**Conditioning**	
100 yd shuttle (in 25 yd increments)	× 6 with 2:30 rest	3-5 mile run	70%-80% MHR

WEEK 3			
Day 1		**Day 2**	
(1) Vertical jump	2 × 5 (SR) 1 × 5 (MR)	(1) Vertical jump	2 × 5 (SR)
		(2a) Deadlift	2 × 5
(2a) DB walking lunge	*1 × 8 each* 4 × 12 each	(2b) Push-up	2 × 10
(2b) Shoulder press	*2 × 5* 4 × 10	**(3) EMOM circuit:**	25 min
(2c) Ab rollout	4 × 12	(a) Deadlift	× 2 @ 74% of ACFT MDL weight
(3a) Pull-up	*2 × 5* 4 × 10	(b) Push-up	15% of ACFT HRP reps
(3b) SB leg curl	4 × 12		
(3c) Front plank	4 × 30 sec		
Conditioning		**Conditioning**	
100 yd shuttle (in 25 yd increments)	× 6 with 2:30 rest	4-6 mile ruck	70%-80% MHR

WEEK 4			
Day 1		**Day 2**	
(1) Vertical jump	2 × 5 (SR) 1 × 5 (MR)	(1) Vertical jump	2 × 5 (SR)
(2a) DB walking lunge	*1 × 8 each* 3 × 12 each	(2a) Deadlift	2 × 5
(2b) Shoulder press	*2 × 5* 3 × 10	(2b) Push-up	2 × 10
(2c) Ab rollout	3 × 12	**(3) EMOM circuit:**	25 min
(3a) Pull-up	*2 × 5* 3 × 10	(a) Deadlift	× 2 @ 74% of ACFT MDL weight
(3b) SB leg curl	3 × 12	(b) Push-up	15% of ACFT HRP reps
(3c) Front plank	3 × 30 sec	(4a) Inverted row	3 × 12
		(4b) Reverse crunch	3 × 12
		(5a) Facepull	3 × 12
		(5b) Side bend	3 × 12 each
Conditioning		**Conditioning**	
100 yd shuttle (in 25 yd increments)	× 6 with 2:30 rest	3-5 mile run	70%-80% MHR

Table 12.3   Two-Day Program, Phase 2

WEEK 1			
Day 1		**Day 2**	
(1) Vertical jump	1 × 5 (SR) 2 × 5 (MR)	(1a) Deadbug arm only	2 × 5 each
(2a) Deadlift	2 × 5 4 × 5	(1b) Deadbug leg only	2 × 5 each
(2b) MB scoop toss	3 × 5	(2) Vertical jump	2 × 5 (SR) 1 × 5 (MR)
(2c) Shoulder press	2 × 5 4 × 5	(3a) RDL	2 × 5 4 × 5 (ECC3)
(3a) Chin-up	2 × 5 4 × 5	(3b) Facepull	4 × 15
(3b) DB forward lunge	1 × 10 each 3 × 15 each	(4) **EMOM circuit:**	20 min
(3c) Ab rollout	3 × 15	(a) Pull-up	× 2
(4a) Lying trunk twist	3 × 8 each	(b) Push-up	× 4
(4b) Band pullapart	3 × 15	(c) Sit-up	× 4
(4c) Wtd plank	3 × 30 sec	(d) Squat	× 4
Conditioning		**Conditioning**	
150 yd shuttle (in 25 yd increments)	× 6 with 2:30 rest	3-5 mile run	75%-85% MHR
WEEK 2			
Day 1		**Day 2**	
(1) Vertical jump	1 × 5 (SR) 2 × 5 (MR)	(1a) Deadbug arm only	2 × 6 each
(2a) Deadlift	2 × 5 5 × 5	(1b) Deadbug leg only	2 × 6 each
(2b) MB scoop toss	3 × 5	(2) Vertical jump	1 × 5 (SR) 2 × 5 (MR)
(2c) Shoulder press	2 × 5 4 × 8	(3a) RDL	2 × 5 4 × 5 (ECC3)
(3a) Chin-up	2 × 5 4 × 8	(3b) Facepull	4 × 15
(3b) DB forward lunge	1 × 10 each 3 × 15 each	(4) **EMOM circuit:**	20 min
(3c) Ab rollout	3 × 15	(a) Pull-up	× 2
(4a) Lying trunk twist	3 × 8 each	(b) Push-up	× 4
(4b) Band pullapart	3 × 15	(c) Sit-up	× 4
(4c) Wtd plank	3 × 30 sec	(d) Squat	× 4
Conditioning		**Conditioning**	
150 yd shuttle (in 25 yd increments)	× 6 with 2:30 rest	3-5 mile run	75%-85% MHR

WEEK 3			
Day 1		**Day 2**	
(1) Vertical jump	1 × 5 (SR) 2 × 5 (MR)	(1) Vertical jump	1 × 5 (SR) 2 × 5 (MR)
(2a) Deadlift	*2 × 5* 5 × 5	(2) **EMOM circuit:**	20 min
(2b) MB scoop toss	3 × 5	(a) Pull-up	× 3
(2c) Shoulder press	*2 × 5* 4 × 8	(b) Push-up	× 5
(3a) Chin-up	*2 × 5* 4 × 8	(c) Sit-up	× 5
(3b) DB forward lunge	*1 × 10 each* 3 × 15 each	(d) Squat	× 7
(3c) Ab rollout	3 × 15		
(4a) Lying trunk twist	3 × 8 each		
(4b) Band pullapart	3 × 15		
(4c) Wtd plank	3 × 30 sec		
Conditioning		**Conditioning**	
150 yd shuttle (in 25 yd increments)	× 6 with 2:30 rest	4-6 mile ruck	75%-85% MHR
WEEK 4			
Day 1		**Day 2**	
(1) Vertical jump	1 × 5 (SR) 2 × 5 (MR)	(1a) Deadbug arm only	2 × 8 each
(2a) Deadlift	*2 × 5* 4 × 5	(1b) Deadbug leg only	2 × 8 each
(2b) MB scoop toss	3 × 5	(2) Vertical jump	1 × 5 (SR) 2 × 5 (MR)
(2c) Shoulder press	*2 × 5* 3 × 8	(3a) RDL	*2 × 5* 3 × 8
(3a) Chin-up	*2 × 5* 3 × 8	(3b) Facepull	4 × 15
(3b) DB forward lunge	*1 × 10 each* 3 × 15 each	(4) **EMOM circuit:**	20 min
(3c) Ab rollout	3 × 15	(a) Pull-up	× 3
(4a) Lying trunk twist	3 × 8 each	(b) Push-up	× 5
(4b) Band pullapart	3 × 15	(c) Sit-up	× 5
(4c) Wtd plank	3 × 30 sec	(d) Squat	× 7
Conditioning		**Conditioning**	
150 yd shuttle (in 25 yd increments)	× 6 with 2:30 rest	3-5 mile run	75%-85% MHR

Table 12.4   Two-Day Program, Phase 3

WEEK 1			
Day 1		**Day 2**	
(1) Lateral bound	3 × 4 each (SR)	(1) Vertical jump	3 × 5 (SR)
(2a) Reverse lunge	*1 × 5 each* 4 × 10 each	(2) MB scoop toss	3 × 5
(2b) DB shoulder press	*1 × 5* 4 × 5	(3) Deadlift	*2 × 5* 4 × 5
(3a) Chin-up	*1 × 5* 4 × 5	(4a) Alt DB prone row	*1 × 5 each* 4 × 10 each
(3b) SA/SL DB RDL	3 × 10 each	(4b) Glute-ham raise	4 × 10
(4a) Rear deltoid raise	3 × 10	(4c) Sit-up	4 × 20
(4b) Ab rollout	3 × 10	(5a) Bench press	*2 × 5* 4 × 5
		(5b) Facepull	4 × 15
		(5c) Pallof press	4 × 5 each side (ECC5)
Conditioning		**Conditioning**	
15 min timed block:	AMRAP	1 mile repeats	× 3 at 2-mile pace with 1:1 W:R ratio
(a) 30 yd Sled push (in 15 yd increments)			
(b) 30 yd DB farmer walk (in 15 yd increments)			
WEEK 2			
Day 1		**Day 2**	
(1) Lateral bound	3 × 4 each (SR)	(1) Vertical jump	3 × 5 (SR)
(2a) Reverse lunge	*1 × 5 each* 4 × 10 each	(2) MB scoop toss	3 × 5
(2b) DB shoulder press	*1 × 5* 4 × 5	(3) Deadlift	*2 × 5* 4 × 5
(3a) Chin-up	*1 × 5* 4 × 5	(4a) Alt DB prone row	*1 × 5 each* 4 × 10 each
(3b) SA/SL DB RDL	3 × 10 each	(4b) Glute-ham raise	4 × 10
(4a) Rear deltoid raise	3 × 10	(4c) Sit-up	4 × 20
(4b) Ab rollout	3 × 10	(5a) Bench press	*2 × 5* 4 × 5
		(5b) Facepull	4 × 15
		(5c) Pallof press	4 × 5 each side (ECC5)
Conditioning		**Conditioning**	
15 min timed block:	AMRAP	1 mile repeats	× 3 at 2-mile pace with 1:1 W:R ratio
(a) 30 yd Sled push (in 15 yd increments)			
(b) 30 yd DB farmer walk (in 15 yd increments)			

WEEK 3			
Day 1		**Day 2**	
(1) Lateral bound	3 × 4 each (SR)	(1) Vertical jump	3 × 5 (SR)
(2a) Reverse lunge	*1 × 5 each* 4 × 8 each	(2) MB scoop toss	3 × 5
(2b) DB shoulder press	*1 × 5* 4 × 3	(3) Deadlift	*2 × 5* 4 × 3
(3a) Chin-up	*1 × 5* 4 × 3	(4a) Alt DB prone row	*1 × 5 each* 4 × 8 each
(3b) SA/SL DB RDL	3 × 8 each	(4b) Glute-ham raise	4 × 10
(4a) Rear deltoid raise	3 × 10	(4c) Sit-up	4 × 25
(4b) Ab rollout	3 × 10	(5a) Bench press	*2 × 5* 4 × 3
		(5b) Facepull	4 × 15
		(5c) Pallof press	4 × 10 each side (ECC3)
Conditioning		**Conditioning**	
15 min timed block:	AMRAP	1 mile repeats	× 3 at 2-mile pace with 1:1 W:R ratio
(a) 30 yd Sled push (in 15 yd increments)			
(b) 30 yd DB farmer walk (in 15 yd increments)			
WEEK 4			
Day 1		**Day 2**	
(1) Lateral bound	3 × 4 each (SR)	(1) Vertical jump	3 × 5 (SR)
(2a) Reverse lunge	*1 × 5 each* 3 × 8 each	(2) MB scoop toss	2 × 5
(2b) DB shoulder press	*1 × 5* 4 × 3	(3) Deadlift	*2 × 5* 4 × 3
(3a) Chin-up	*1 × 5* 4 × 3	(4a) Alt DB prone row	*1 × 5 each* 3 × 8 each
(3b) SA/SL DB RDL	3 × 8 each	(4b) Glute-ham raise	3 × 10
(4a) Rear deltoid raise	3 × 10	(4c) Sit-up	3 × 25
(4b) Ab rollout	3 × 10	(5a) Bench press	*2 × 5* 4 × 3
		(5b) Facepull	4 × 15
		(5c) Pallof press	4 × 10 each side (ECC3)
Conditioning		**Conditioning**	
15 min timed block:	AMRAP	1 mile repeats	× 3 at 2-mile pace with 1:1 W:R ratio
(a) 30 yd Sled push (in 15 yd increments)			
(b) 30 yd DB farmer walk (in 15 yd increments)			

Table 12.5   Two-Day Program, Phase 4

WEEK 1			
Day 1		**Day 2**	
(1) Lateral bound	1 × 4 each (SR) 2 × 4 each (MR)	(1) Vertical jump	1 × 5 (SR) 2 × 5 (MR)
(2) DB quarter squat jump	*1 × 5 (SR)* 2 × 5 (SR)	(2) Tuck jump	2 × 5 (MR)
(3a) Pull-up	*1 × 5* 4 × 5	(3a) Deadlift	*2 × 5* 4 × 5
(3b) DB forward lunge	*1 × 5 each* 4 × 10 each	(3b) MB scoop toss	4 × 5
(4a) Wtd push-up	*1 × 10* 4 × 10	(4a) DB prone row	*1 × 5* 4 × 10
(4b) DB SL RDL	3 × 10 each	(4b) Poor man's glute-ham raise	4 × 5
(5a) Facepull	3 × 15	(5a) Bench press	*2 × 5* 4 × 5
(5b) Hanging knee raise	3 × 12	(5b) RG band pullapart	4 × 15
		(5c) Ab rollout	3 × 12
Conditioning		**Conditioning**	
150 yd shuttle (in 25 yd increments)	× 5 with 1:30 rest	400 m repeats	× 9 at 5%-15% faster than 2-mile pace with 1:1 W:R ratio
WEEK 2			
Day 1		**Day 2**	
(1) Lateral bound	1 × 4 each (SR) 2 × 4 each (MR)	(1) Vertical jump	1 × 5 (SR) 2 × 5 (MR)
(2) DB quarter squat jump	*1 × 5 (SR)* 2 × 5 (SR)	(2) Tuck jump	2 × 5 (MR)
(3a) Pull-up	*1 × 5* 4 × 5	(3a) Deadlift	*2 × 5* 4 × 3
(3b) DB forward lunge	*1 × 5 each* 4 × 10 each	(3b) MB scoop toss	3 × 5
(4a) Wtd push-up	*1 × 10* 4 × 10	(4a) DB prone row	*1 × 5* 4 × 8
(4b) DB SL RDL	3 × 10 each	(4b) Poor man's glute-ham raise	4 × 5
(5a) Facepull	3 × 15	(5a) Bench press	*2 × 5* 4 × 3
(5b) Hanging knee raise	3 × 12	(5b) RG band pullapart	4 × 15
		(5c) Ab rollout	3 × 12
Conditioning		**Conditioning**	
150 yd shuttle (in 25 yd increments)	× 5 with 1:30 rest	400 m repeats	× 9 at 5%-15% faster than 2-mile pace with 1:1 W:R ratio

WEEK 3			
Day 1		**Day 2**	
(1) Lateral bound	1 × 4 each (SR) 2 × 4 each (MR)	(1) Vertical jump	1 × 5 (SR) 2 × 5 (MR)
(2) DB quarter squat jump	*1 × 5 (SR)* 2 × 5 (SR)	(2) Tuck jump	2 × 5 (MR)
(3a) Pull-up	*1 × 5* 4 × 3,2,2,2	(3a) Deadlift	*2 × 5* 4 × 3
(3b) DB forward lunge	*1 × 5 each* 4 × 8 each	(3b) MB scoop toss	3 × 5
(4a) Wtd push-up	*1 × 10* 4 × 8	(4a) DB prone row	*1 × 5* 4 × 8
(4b) DB SL RDL	3 × 8 each	(4b) Poor man's glute-ham raise	4 × 6
(5a) Facepull	3 × 15	(5a) Bench press	*2 × 5* 4 × 3,2,1,1
(5b) Hanging knee raise	3 × 15	(5b) RG band pullapart	4 × 15
		(5c) Ab rollout	3 × 15
Conditioning		**Conditioning**	
150 yd shuttle (in 25 yd increments)	× 5 with 1:30 rest	3-5 mile run	75%-85% MHR
WEEK 4			
Day 1		**Day 2**	
(1) Lateral bound	1 × 4 each (SR) 2 × 4 each (MR)	(1) Vertical jump	1 × 5 (SR) 2 × 5 (MR)
(2) DB quarter squat jump	*1 × 5 (SR)* 2 × 5 (SR)	(2) Tuck jump	2 × 5 (MR)
(3a) Pull-up	*1 × 5* 3 × 3	(3a) Deadlift	*2 × 5* 4 × 3,2,1,1
(3b) DB forward lunge	*1 × 5 each* 3 × 8 each	(3b) MB scoop toss	2 × 4
(4a) Wtd push-up	*1 × 10* 3 × 8	(4a) DB prone row	*1 × 5* 3 × 8
(4b) DB SL RDL	3 × 8 each	(4b) Poor man's glute-ham raise	3 × 5
(5a) Facepull	3 × 15	(5a) Bench press	*2 × 5* 4 × 3
(5b) Hanging knee raise	3 × 15	(5b) RG band pullapart	4 × 15
		(5c) Ab rollout	3 × 15
Conditioning		**Conditioning**	
150 yd shuttle (in 25 yd increments)	× 5 with 1:30 rest	400 m repeats	× 9 at 5%-15% faster than 2-mile pace with 1:1 W:R ratio

Table 12.6   Two-Day Program, Phase 5

WEEK 1			
Day 1		**Day 2**	
(1) Lateral bound	1 × 4 each (SR) 2 × 4 each (MR)	(1) Vertical jump	1 × 5 (SR) 2 × 5 (MR)
(2) MB scoop toss	3 × 5	(2) DB quarter squat jump	1 × 5 (MR) 1 × 5 (MR)
(3) Deadlift	2 × 5 6 × 5,3,1,5,3,1	(3) Squat	2 × 5 4 × 5
(4a) Pull-up (working sets: Wtd pull-up)	1 × 5 Work up to a 5RM then do 2 × 8 @ 80% of 5RM	(4a) RG bent-over row	1 × 5 4 × 5
(4b) Glute-ham raise	4 × 10	(4b) Push-up on DBs	1 × 10% of ACFT HRP reps 4 × 50% of ACFT HRP reps
(5a) Shoulder press	2 × 5 Work up to a 5RM then do 2 × 8 @ 80% of 5RM	(5a) SL RDL	3 × 8 each
(5b) RG band pullapart	4 × 15	(5b) Facepull	3 × 15
(5c) Leg tuck	4 × 5-10	(5c) Roman side crunch	3 × 10 each
Conditioning		**Conditioning**	
Backward sled drag (25 yds) + shuttle (25 yds)	× 6 with 1:3 W:R ratio	800 m repeats	× 5 at 5%-15% faster than 2-mile pace with 1:1 W:R ratio
WEEK 2			
Day 1		**Day 2**	
(1) Lateral bound	1 × 4 each (SR) 2 × 4 each (MR)	(1) Vertical jump	1 × 5 (SR) 2 × 5 (MR)
(2) MB scoop toss	3 × 5	(2) DB quarter squat jump	1 × 5 (MR) 1 × 5 (MR)
(3) Deadlift	2 × 5 6 × 5,3,1,5,3,1	(3) Squat	2 × 5 4 × 5
(4a) Pull-up (working sets: Wtd pull-up)	1 × 5 Work up to a 5RM then do 2 × 8 @ 80% of 5RM	(4a) RG bent-over row	1 × 5 4 × 5
(4b) Glute-ham raise	4 × 10	(4b) Push-up on DBs	1 × 10% of ACFT HRP reps 4 × 50% of ACFT HRP reps
(5a) Shoulder press	2 × 5 Work up to a 5RM then do 2 × 8 @ 80% of 5RM	(5a) SL RDL	3 × 8 each
(5b) RG band pullapart	4 × 15	(5b) Facepull	3 × 15
(5c) Leg tuck	4 × 5-10	(5c) Roman side crunch	3 × 10 each
Conditioning		**Conditioning**	
Backward sled drag (25 yds) + shuttle (25 yds)	× 6 with 1:3 W:R ratio	800 m repeats	× 5 at 5%-15% faster than 2-mile pace with 1:1 W:R ratio

WEEK 3			
Day 1		**Day 2**	
(1) Lateral bound	1 × 4 each (SR) 2 × 4 each (MR)	(1) Vertical jump	1 × 5 (SR) 2 × 5 (MR)
(2) MB scoop toss	3 × 5	(2) DB quarter squat jump	*1 × 5 (MR)* 1 × 5 (MR)
(3) Deadlift	*2 × 5* Work up to a 3RM	(3) Squat	*2 × 5* 4 × 5
(4a) Pull-up (working sets: Wtd pull-up)	*1 × 5* Work up to a 3RM then do 2 × 6 @ 80% of 3RM	(4a) RG bent-over row	*1 × 5* 4 × 4
(4b) Glute-ham raise	4 × 10	(4b) Push-up on DBs	*1 × 10% of ACFT HRP reps* 4 × 60% of ACFT HRP reps
(5a) Shoulder press	*2 × 5* Work up to a 3RM then do 2 × 6 @ 80% of 3RM	(5a) SL RDL	3 × 8 each
(5b) RG band pullapart	4 × 15	(5b) Facepull	3 × 15
(5c) Leg tuck	4 × 5-10	(5c) Roman side crunch	3 × 15 each
Conditioning		**Conditioning**	
Backward sled drag (25 yds) + shuttle (25 yds)	× 6 with 1:3 W:R ratio	3-5 mile run	75%-85% MHR
WEEK 4			
Day 1		**Day 2**	
(1) Lateral bound	1 × 4 each (SR) 2 × 4 each (MR)	(1) Vertical jump	1 × 5 (SR) 2 × 5 (MR)
(2) MB scoop toss	3 × 5	(2) DB quarter squat jump	*1 × 5 (MR)* 1 × 5 (MR)
(3) Deadlift	*2 × 5* 3 × 3	(3) Squat	*2 × 5* 3 × 5
(4a) Pull-up	*2 × 5* 3 × 3	(4a) RG bent-over row	*1 × 5* 3 × 5
(4b) Glute-ham raise	3 × 10	(4b) Push-up on DBs	*1 × 10% of ACFT HRP reps* 3 × 60% of ACFT HRP reps
(5a) Shoulder press	*2 × 5* 3 × 3	(5a) SL RDL	3 × 8 each
(5b) RG band pullapart	4 × 15	(5b) Facepull	3 × 15
(5c) Leg tuck	4 × 5-10	(5c) Roman side crunch	3 × 15 each
Conditioning		**Conditioning**	
Backward sled drag (25 yds) + shuttle (25 yds)	× 6 with 1:3 W:R ratio	1 mile time trial	Rest 10 minutes
		800 m repeats	× 2 at 5%-15% faster than 2-mile pace with 1:1 W:R ratio

Table 12.7 Two-Day Program, Phase 6

WEEK 1			
Day 1		**Day 2**	
(1) Lateral bound	1 × 4 each (SR) 2 × 4 each (MR)	(1) High ankle hop	1 × 10 (MR)
(2) 50 yd shuttle with alt foot plant	× 6	(2) Vertical jump	1 × 5 (SR)
(3) MB scoop toss	3 × 5	(3) Power skip	2 × 4 each
(4a) Chin-up	2 × 5 4 × 8,8,6,6 1 × AMRAP (>5 reps)	(4) ACFT practice	90% of previous ACFT results
(4b) RFE DB SA split squat	1 × 5 each 4 × 10 each		
(5a) Incline bench press	2 × 5 4 × 8,8,6,6		
(5b) RDL	1 × 5 3 × 5 1 × 10		
(6a) Leg tuck	4 × 5-20		
(6b) Facepull	4 × 15		
Conditioning		**Conditioning**	
400 m repeats	× 9 at 5%-15% faster than 1-mile pace with 1:1 W:R ratio	None	
WEEK 2			
Day 1		**Day 2**	
(1) Lateral bound	1 × 4 each (SR) 2 × 4 each (MR)	(1) High ankle hop	1 × 10 (MR)
(2) 50 yd shuttle with alt foot plant	× 6	(2) Vertical jump	1 × 5 (SR)
(3) MB scoop toss	3 × 5	(3) Power skip	2 × 4 each
(4a) Chin-up	2 × 5 4 × 8,8,6,6 1 × AMRAP (>5 reps)	(4) ACFT practice	100% of previous ACFT results
(4b) RFE DB SA split squat	1 × 5 each 4 × 10 each		
(5a) Incline bench press	2 × 5 4 × 8,8,6,6		
(5b) RDL	1 × 5 3 × 5 1 × 10		
(6a) Leg tuck	4 × 5-20		
(6b) Facepull	4 × 15		
Conditioning		**Conditioning**	
400 m repeats	× 9 at 5%-15% faster than 1-mile pace with 1:1 W:R ratio	None	

WEEK 3			
Day 1		**Day 2**	
(1) Lateral bound	1 × 4 each (SR) 2 × 4 each (MR)	(1) High ankle hop	1 × 10 (MR)
(2) 50 yd shuttle with alt foot plant	× 6	(2) Vertical jump	1 × 5 (SR)
(3) MB scoop toss	3 × 5	(3) Power skip	2 × 4 each
(4a) Chin-up	2 × 5 3 × 5	(4) ACFT practice	Practice ACFT (all-out)
(4b) RFE DB SA split squat	1 × 5 each 3 × 10 each		
(5a) Incline bench press	2 × 5 3 × 5		
(5b) RDL	1 × 5 3 × 5		
(6a) Leg tuck	4 × 5-20		
(6b) Facepull	4 × 15		
Conditioning		**Conditioning**	
400 m repeats	× 9 at 5%-15% faster than 1-mile pace with 1:1 W:R ratio	None	

WEEK 4			
Day 1		**Day 2**	
(1) Lateral bound	1 × 4 each (SR) 1 × 4 each (MR)	(1) High ankle hop	1 × 10 (MR)
(2) 50 yd shuttle with alt foot plant	× 4	(2) Vertical jump	1 × 5 (SR)
(3) MB scoop toss	3 × 5	(3) Power skip	2 × 4 each
(4a) Chin-up	2 × 5 3 × 5	(4) ACFT practice	80% of last week's ACFT results
(4b) RFE DB SA split squat	1 × 5 each 3 × 6 each		
(5a) Incline bench press	2 × 5 3 × 5		
(5b) RDL	1 × 5 3 × 5		
(6a) Leg tuck	2 × 5-20		
(6b) Facepull	2 × 15		
Conditioning		**Conditioning**	
2 mile run	75%-85% MHR	None	

Table 12.8   Three-Day Program, Phase 1

WEEK 1					
Day 1		**Day 2**		**Day 3**	
(1) Vertical jump	2 × 5 (SR)	(1) Vertical jump	2 × 5 (SR)	(1) High ankle hop	2 × 10 (MR)
(2a) DB walking lunge	*1 × 8 each* 3 × 12 each	(2a) Deadlift	2 × 5	(2) Power skip	2 × 4 each
(2b) Shoulder press	*2 × 5* 3 × 10	(2b) Push-up	2 × 10	(3) 40 yd build-ups	× 4
(2c) Ab rollout	3 × 12	(3) **EMOM circuit:**	15 min		
(3a) Pull-up	*2 × 5* 3 × 10	(a) Deadlift	× 2 @ 74% of ACFT MDL weight		
(3b) SB leg curl	3 × 12	(b) Push-up	15% of ACFT HRP reps		
(3c) Front plank	3 × 30 sec	(4a) Inverted row	3 × 12		
		(4b) Reverse crunch	3 × 12		
		(5a) Facepull	3 × 12		
		(5b) Side bend	3 × 12 each		
Conditioning		**Conditioning**		**Conditioning**	
100 yd shuttle (in 25 yd increments)	× 6 with 2:30 rest	None		3-5 mile run	70%-80% MHR
WEEK 2					
Day 1		**Day 2**		**Day 3**	
(1) Vertical jump	2 × 5 (SR)	(1) Vertical jump	2 × 5 (SR)	(1) High ankle hop	2 × 10 (MR)
(2a) DB walking lunge	*1 × 8 each* 3 × 12 each	(2a) Deadlift	2 × 5	(2) Power skip	2 × 4 each
(2b) Shoulder press	*2 × 5* 3 × 10	(2b) Push-up	2 × 10		
(2c) Ab rollout	3 × 12	(3) **EMOM circuit:**	20 min		
(3a) Pull-up	*2 × 5* 3 × 10	(a) Deadlift	× 2 @ 74% of ACFT MDL weight		
(3b) SB leg curl	3 × 12	(b) Push-up	15% of ACFT HRP reps		
(3c) Front plank	3 × 30 sec	(4a) Inverted row	3 × 12		
		(4b) Reverse crunch	3 × 12		
		(5a) Facepull	3 × 12		
		(5b) Side bend	3 × 12 each		
Conditioning		**Conditioning**		**Conditioning**	
100 yd shuttle (in 25 yd increments)	× 6 with 2:30 rest	None		5-6 mile ruck	70%-80% MHR

WEEK 3					
Day 1		**Day 2**		**Day 3**	
(1) Vertical jump	2 × 5 (SR) 1 × 5 (MR)	(1) Vertical jump	2 × 5 (SR)	(1) High ankle hop	2 × 10 (MR)
(2a) DB walking lunge	*1 × 8 each* 4 × 12 each	(2a) Deadlift	2 × 5	(2) Power skip	2 × 4 each
(2b) Shoulder press	*2 × 5* 4 × 10	(2b) Push-up	2 × 10	(3) 40 yd build-ups	× 4
(2c) Ab rollout	4 × 12	(3) **EMOM circuit:**	25 min		
(3a) Pull-up	*2 × 5* 4 × 10	(a) Deadlift	× 2 @ 74% of ACFT MDL weight		
(3b) SB leg curl	4 × 12	(b) Push-up	15% of ACFT HRP reps		
(3c) Front plank	4 × 30 sec	(4a) Inverted row	4 × 12		
		(4b) Reverse crunch	4 × 15		
		(5a) Facepull	4 × 12		
		(5b) Side bend	4 × 12 each		
Conditioning		**Conditioning**		**Conditioning**	
100 yd shuttle (in 25 yd increments)	× 6 with 2:30 rest	None		3-5 mile run	70%-80% MHR
WEEK 4					
Day 1		**Day 2**		**Day 3**	
(1) Vertical jump	2 × 5 (SR) 1 × 5 (MR)	(1) Vertical jump	2 × 5 (SR)	(1) High ankle hop	2 × 10 (MR)
(2a) DB walking lunge	*1 × 8 each* 3 × 12 each	(2a) Deadlift	2 × 5	(2) Power skip	2 × 4 each
(2b) Shoulder press	*2 × 5* 3 × 10	(2b) Push-up	2 × 10		
(2c) Ab rollout	3 × 12	(3) **EMOM circuit:**	25 min		
(3a) Pull-up	*2 × 5* 3 × 10	(a) Deadlift	× 2 @ 74% of ACFT MDL weight		
(3b) SB leg curl	3 × 12	(b) Push-up	15% of ACFT HRP reps		
(3c) Front plank	3 × 30 sec	(4a) Inverted row	3 × 12		
		(4b) Reverse crunch	3 × 12		
		(5a) Facepull	3 × 12		
		(5b) Side bend	3 × 12 each		
Conditioning		**Conditioning**		**Conditioning**	
100 yd shuttle (in 25 yd increments)	× 6 with 2:30 rest	None		5-6 mile ruck	70%-80% MHR

Table 12.9   Three-Day Program, Phase 2

WEEK 1					
Day 1		**Day 2**		**Day 3**	
(1) Vertical jump	1 × 5 (SR) 2 × 5 (MR)	(1a) Deadbug arm only	2 × 5 each	(1) High ankle hop	2 × 10 (MR)
(2a) Deadlift	2 × 5 4 × 5	(1b) Deadbug leg only	2 × 5 each	(2) Power skip	2 × 4 each
(2b) MB scoop toss	3 × 5	(2) Vertical jump	2 × 5 (SR) 1 × 5 (MR)	(3) 40 yd build-ups	× 6
(2c) Shoulder press	2 × 5 4 × 5	(3a) RDL	2 × 5 4 × 5 (ECC3)		
(3a) Chin-up	2 × 5 4 × 5	(3b) Facepull	4 × 15		
(3b) DB forward lunge	1 × 10 each 3 × 15 each	(4) **EMOM circuit:**	20 min		
(3c) Ab rollout	3 × 15	(a) Pull-up	× 2		
(4a) Lying trunk twist	3 × 8 each	(b) Push-up	× 4		
(4b) Band pull-apart	3 × 15	(c) Sit-up	× 4		
(4c) Wtd plank	3 × 30 sec	(d) Squat	× 4		
Conditioning		**Conditioning**		**Conditioning**	
150 yd shuttle (in 25 yd increments)	× 6 with 2:30 rest	Fan bike	4 × 30 sec with 4 min rest	3-5 mile run	75%-85% MHR
WEEK 2					
Day 1		**Day 2**		**Day 3**	
(1) Vertical jump	1 × 5 (SR) 2 × 5 (MR)	(1a) Deadbug arm only	2 × 6 each	(1) High ankle hop	2 × 10 (MR)
(2a) Deadlift	2 × 5 5 × 5	(1b) Deadbug leg only	2 × 6 each	(2) Power skip	2 × 4 each
(2b) MB scoop toss	3 × 5	(2) Vertical jump	1 × 5 (SR) 2 × 5 (MR)	(3) 40 yd build-ups	× 6
(2c) Shoulder press	2 × 5 4 × 8	(3a) RDL	2 × 5 4 × 5 (ECC3)		
(3a) Chin-up	2 × 5 4 × 8	(3b) Facepull	4 × 15		
(3b) DB forward lunge	1 × 10 each 3 × 15 each	(4) **EMOM circuit:**	20 min		
(3c) Ab rollout	3 × 15	(a) Pull-up	× 2		
(4a) Lying trunk twist	3 × 8 each	(b) Push-up	× 4		
(4b) Band pull-apart	3 × 15	(c) Sit-up	× 4		
(4c) Wtd plank	3 × 30 sec	(d) Squat	× 4		
Conditioning		**Conditioning**		**Conditioning**	
150 yd shuttle (in 25 yd increments)	× 6 with 2:30 rest	Fan bike	4 × 30 sec with 4 min rest	3-5 mile run	75%-85% MHR

Three-Day Program, Phase 2

WEEK 3					
Day 1		**Day 2**		**Day 3**	
(1) Vertical jump	1 × 5 (SR) 2 × 5 (MR)	(1a) Deadbug arm only	2 × 8 each	(1) High ankle hop	2 × 10 (MR)
(2a) Deadlift	2 × 5 5 × 5	(1b) Deadbug leg only	2 × 8 each	(2) Power skip	2 × 4 each
(2b) MB scoop toss	3 × 5	(2) Vertical jump	1 × 5 (SR) 2 × 5 (MR)	(3) 40 yd build-ups	× 6
(2c) Shoulder press	2 × 5 4 × 8	(3a) RDL	2 × 5 4 × 5 (ECC3)		
(3a) Chin-up	2 × 5 4 × 8	(3b) Facepull	4 × 15		
(3b) DB forward lunge	1 × 10 each 3 × 15 each	(4) **EMOM circuit:**	20 min		
(3c) Ab rollout	3 × 15	(a) Pull-up	× 3		
(4a) Lying trunk twist	3 × 8 each	(b) Push-up	× 5		
(4b) Band pull-apart	3 × 15	(c) Sit-up	× 5		
(4c) Wtd plank	3 × 30 sec	(d) Squat	× 7		
Conditioning		**Conditioning**		**Conditioning**	
150 yd shuttle (in 25 yd increments)	× 6 with 2:30 rest	Fan bike	4 × 30 sec with 3 min rest	5-6 mile ruck	75%-85% MHR
WEEK 4					
Day 1		**Day 2**		**Day 3**	
(1) Vertical jump	1 × 5 (SR) 2 × 5 (MR)	(1a) Deadbug arm only	2 × 8 each	(1) High ankle hop	2 × 10 (MR)
(2a) Deadlift	2 × 5 4 × 5	(1b) Deadbug leg only	2 × 8 each	(2) Power skip	2 × 4 each
(2b) MB scoop toss	3 × 5	(2) Vertical jump	1 × 5 (SR) 2 × 5 (MR)	(3) 40 yd build-ups	× 6
(2c) Shoulder press	2 × 5 3 × 8	(3a) RDL	2 × 5 3 × 8		
(3a) Chin-up	2 × 5 3 × 8	(3b) Facepull	4 × 15		
(3b) DB forward lunge	1 × 10 each 3 × 15 each	(4) **EMOM circuit:**	20 min		
(3c) Ab rollout	3 × 15	(a) Pull-up	× 3		
(4a) Lying trunk twist	3 × 8 each	(b) Push-up	× 5		
(4b) Band pull-apart	3 × 15	(c) Sit-up	× 5		
(4c) Wtd plank	3 × 30 sec	(d) Squat	× 7		
Conditioning		**Conditioning**		**Conditioning**	
150 yd shuttle (in 25 yd increments)	× 6 with 2:30 rest	Fan bike	4 × 30 sec with 3 min rest	3-5 mile run	75%-85% MHR

Table 12.10   Three-Day Program, Phase 3

WEEK 1					
Day 1		**Day 2**		**Day 3**	
(1) Lateral bound	3 × 4 each (SR)	(1) Vertical jump	3 × 5 (SR)	(1) High ankle hop	2 × 10 (MR)
(2a) Reverse lunge	*1 × 5 each* 4 × 10 each	(2) MB scoop toss	3 × 5	(2) Power skip	2 × 4 each
(2b) DB shoulder press	*1 × 5* 4 × 5	(3) Deadlift	*2 × 5* 4 × 5	(3) 40 yd build-ups	× 6
(3a) Chin-up	*1 × 5* 4 × 5	(4a) Alt DB prone row	*1 × 5 each* 4 × 10 each		
(3b) SA/SL DB RDL	3 × 10 each	(4b) Glute-ham raise	4 × 10		
(4a) Rear deltoid raise	3 × 10	(4c) Sit-up	4 × 20		
(4b) Ab rollout	3 × 10	(5a) Bench press	*2 × 5* 4 × 5		
		(5b) Facepull	4 × 15		
		(5c) Pallof press	4 × 5 each side (ECC5)		
Conditioning		**Conditioning**		**Conditioning**	
Rower time trial	500 m × 3 with 5 min rest	**15 min timed block:**	AMRAP	1 mile repeats	× 3 at 2-mile pace with 1:1 W:R ratio
		(a) 30 yd Sled push (in 15 yd increments)			
		(b) 30 yd DB farmer walk (in 15 yd increments)			
WEEK 2					
Day 1		**Day 2**		**Day 3**	
(1) Lateral bound	3 × 4 each (SR)	(1) Vertical jump	3 × 5 (SR)	(1) High ankle hop	2 × 10 (MR)
(2a) Reverse lunge	*1 × 5 each* 4 × 10 each	(2) MB scoop toss	3 × 5	(2) Power skip	2 × 4 each
(2b) DB shoulder press	*1 × 5* 4 × 5	(3) Deadlift	*2 × 5* 4 × 5	(3) 40 yd build-ups	× 6
(3a) Chin-up	*1 × 5* 4 × 5	(4a) Alt DB prone row	*1 × 5 each* 4 × 10 each		
(3b) SA/SL DB RDL	3 × 10 each	(4b) Glute-ham raise	4 × 10		
(4a) Rear deltoid raise	3 × 10	(4c) Sit-up	4 × 20		
(4b) Ab rollout	3 × 10	(5a) Bench press	*2 × 5* 4 × 5		
		(5b) Facepull	4 × 15		
		(5c) Pallof press	4 × 5 each side (ECC5)		
Conditioning		**Conditioning**		**Conditioning**	
Rower time trial	500 m × 3 with 5 min rest	**15 min timed block:**	AMRAP	1 mile repeats	× 3 at 2-mile pace with 1:1 W:R ratio
		(a) 30 yd Sled push (in 15 yd increments)			
		(b) 30 yd DB farmer walk (in 15 yd increments)			

Three-Day Program, Phase 3

WEEK 3					
Day 1		**Day 2**		**Day 3**	
(1) Lateral bound	3 × 4 each (SR)	(1) Vertical jump	3 × 5 (SR)	(1) High ankle hop	2 × 10 (MR)
(2a) Reverse lunge	*1 × 5 each* 4 × 8 each	(2) MB scoop toss	3 × 5	(2) Power skip	2 × 4 each
(2b) DB shoulder press	*1 × 5* 4 × 3	(3) Deadlift	*2 × 5* 4 × 3	(3) 40 yd build-ups	× 6
(3a) Chin-up	*1 × 5* 4 × 3	(4a) Alt DB prone row	*1 × 5 each* 4 × 8 each		
(3b) SA/SL DB RDL	3 × 8 each	(4b) Glute-ham raise	4 × 10		
(4a) Rear deltoid raise	3 × 10	(4c) Sit-up	4 × 25		
(4b) Ab rollout	3 × 10	(5a) Bench press	*2 × 5* 4 × 3		
		(5b) Facepull	4 × 15		
		(5c) Pallof press	4 × 10 each side (ECC3)		
Conditioning		**Conditioning**		**Conditioning**	
Rower time trial	500 m × 3 with 5 min rest	**15 min timed block:**	AMRAP	1 mile repeats	× 3 at 2-mile pace with 1:1 W:R ratio
		(a) 30 yd Sled push (in 15 yd increments)			
		(b) 30 yd DB farmer walk (in 15 yd increments)			
WEEK 4					
Day 1		**Day 2**		**Day 3**	
(1) Lateral bound	3 × 4 each (SR)	(1) Vertical jump	3 × 5 (SR)	(1) High ankle hop	2 × 10 (MR)
(2a) Reverse lunge	*1 × 5 each* 3 × 8 each	(2) MB scoop toss	2 × 5	(2) Power skip	2 × 4 each
(2b) DB shoulder press	*1 × 5* 4 × 3	(3) Deadlift	*2 × 5* 4 × 3	(3) 40 yd build-ups	× 6
(3a) Chin-up	*1 × 5* 4 × 3	(4a) Alt DB prone row	*1 × 5 each* 3 × 8 each		
(3b) SA/SL DB RDL	3 × 8 each	(4b) Glute-ham raise	3 × 10		
(4a) Rear deltoid raise	3 × 10	(4c) Sit-up	3 × 25		
(4b) Ab rollout	3 × 10	(5a) Bench press	*2 × 5* 4 × 3		
		(5b) Facepull	4 × 15		
		(5c) Pallof press	4 × 10 each side (ECC3)		
Conditioning		**Conditioning**		**Conditioning**	
Rower time trial	500 m × 3 with 5 min rest	**15 min timed block:**	AMRAP	1 mile repeats	× 3 at 2-mile pace with 1:1 W:R ratio
		(a) 30 yd Sled push (in 15 yd increments)			
		(b) 30 yd DB farmer walk (in 15 yd increments)			

Table 12.11 Three-Day Program, Phase 4

WEEK 1					
Day 1		**Day 2**		**Day 3**	
(1) Lateral bound	1 × 4 each (SR) 2 × 4 each (MR)	(1) Vertical jump	1 × 5 (SR) 2 × 5 (MR)	(1) High ankle hop	2 × 10 (MR)
(2) DB quarter squat jump	1 × 5 (SR) 2 × 5 (SR)	(2) Tuck jump	2 × 5 (MR)	(2) Bound	2 × 4 each (SR)
(3a) Pull-up	1 × 5 4 × 5	(3a) Deadlift	2 × 5 4 × 5	(3) Power skip	2 × 4 each
(3b) DB forward lunge	1 × 5 each 4 × 10 each	(3b) MB scoop toss	4 × 5	(4) 40 yd build-ups	× 6
(4a) Wtd push-up	1 × 10 4 × 10	(4a) DB prone row	1 × 5 4 × 10		
(4b) DB SL RDL	3 × 10 each	(4b) Poor man's glute-ham raise	4 × 5		
(5a) Facepull	3 × 15	(5a) Bench press	2 × 5 4 × 5		
(5b) Hanging knee raise	3 × 12	(5b) RG band pull-apart	4 × 15		
		(5c) Ab rollout	3 × 12		
Conditioning		**Conditioning**		**Conditioning**	
150 yd shuttle (in 25 yd increments)	× 5 with 1:30 rest	8 rounds for time:		400 m repeats	× 9 at 5%-15% faster than 2-mile pace with 1:1 W:R ratio
		(a) Fan bike	15 calories		
		(b) Hand release push-up	× 10		
WEEK 2					
Day 1		**Day 2**		**Day 3**	
(1) Lateral bound	1 × 4 each (SR) 2 × 4 each (MR)	(1) Vertical jump	1 × 5 (SR) 2 × 5 (MR)	(1) High ankle hop	2 × 10 (MR)
(2) DB quarter squat jump	1 × 5 (SR) 2 × 5 (SR)	(2) Tuck jump	2 × 5 (MR)	(2) Bound	2 × 4 each (SR)
(3a) Pull-up	1 × 5 4 × 5	(3a) Deadlift	2 × 5 4 × 3	(3) Power skip	2 × 4 each
(3b) DB forward lunge	1 × 5 each 4 × 10 each	(3b) MB scoop toss	3 × 5	(4) 40 yd build-ups	× 6
(4a) Wtd push-up	1 × 10 4 × 10	(4a) DB prone row	1 × 5 4 × 8		
(4b) DB SL RDL	3 × 10 each	(4b) Poor man's glute-ham raise	4 × 5		
(5a) Facepull	3 × 15	(5a) Bench press	2 × 5 4 × 3		
(5b) Hanging knee raise	3 × 12	(5b) RG band pull-apart	4 × 15		
		(5c) Ab rollout	3 × 12		
Conditioning		**Conditioning**		**Conditioning**	
150 yd shuttle (in 25 yd increments)	× 5 with 1:30 rest	8 rounds for time:		400 m repeats	× 9 at 5%-15% faster than 2-mile pace with 1:1 W:R ratio
		(a) Fan bike	15 calories		
		(b) Hand release push-up	× 10		

WEEK 3					
Day 1		**Day 2**		**Day 3**	
(1) Lateral bound	1 × 4 each (SR) 2 × 4 each (MR)	(1) Vertical jump	1 × 5 (SR) 2 × 5 (MR)	(1) High ankle hop	2 × 10 (MR)
(2) DB quarter squat jump	*1 × 5 (SR)* 2 × 5 (SR)	(2) Tuck jump	2 × 5 (MR)	(2) Bound	2 × 4 each (SR)
(3a) Pull-up	*1 × 5* 4 × 3,2,2,2	(3a) Deadlift	*2 × 5* 4 × 3	(3) Power skip	2 × 4 each
(3b) DB forward lunge	*1 × 5 each* 4 × 8 each	(3b) MB scoop toss	3 × 5	(4) 40 yd build-ups	× 6
(4a) Wtd push-up	*1 × 10* 4 × 8	(4a) DB prone row	*1 × 5* 4 × 8		
(4b) DB SL RDL	3 × 8 each	(4b) Poor man's glute-ham raise	4 × 6		
(5a) Facepull	3 × 15	(5a) Bench press	*2 × 5* 4 × 3,2,1,1		
(5b) Hanging knee raise	3 × 15	(5b) RG band pull-apart	4 × 15		
		(5c) Ab rollout	3 × 15		
Conditioning		**Conditioning**		**Conditioning**	
150 yd shuttle (in 25 yd increments)	× 5 with 1:30 rest	Rower time trial	500 m × 3 with 1:3 W:R ratio	3-5 mile run	75%-85% MHR
WEEK 4					
Day 1		**Day 2**		**Day 3**	
(1) Lateral bound	1 × 4 each (SR) 2 × 4 each (MR)	(1) Vertical jump	1 × 5 (SR) 2 × 5 (MR)	(1) High ankle hop	2 × 10 (MR)
(2) DB quarter squat jump	*1 × 5 (SR)* 2 × 5 (SR)	(2) Tuck jump	2 × 5 (MR)	(2) Bound	2 × 4 each (SR)
(3a) Pull-up	*1 × 5* 3 × 3	(3a) Deadlift	*2 × 5* 4 × 3,2,1,1	(3) Power skip	2 × 4 each
(3b) DB forward lunge	*1 × 5 each* 3 × 8 each	(3b) MB scoop toss	2 × 4	(4) 40 yd build-ups	× 6
(4a) Wtd push-up	*1 × 10* 3 × 8	(4a) DB prone row	*1 × 5* 3 × 8		
(4b) DB SL RDL	3 × 8 each	(4b) Poor man's glute-ham raise	3 × 5		
(5a) Facepull	3 × 15	(5a) Bench press	*2 × 5* 4 × 3		
(5b) Hanging knee raise	3 × 15	(5b) RG band pull-apart	4 × 15		
		(5c) Ab rollout	3 × 15		
Conditioning		**Conditioning**		**Conditioning**	
150 yd shuttle (in 25 yd increments)	× 5 with 1:30 rest	**8 rounds for time:**		400 m repeats	× 9 at 5%-15% faster than 2-mile pace with 1:1 W:R ratio
		(a) Fan bike	15 calories		
		(b) Hand release push-up	× 10		

Table 12.12   Three-Day Program, Phase 5

WEEK 1					
Day 1		**Day 2**		**Day 3**	
(1) Lateral bound	1 × 4 each (SR) 2 × 4 each (MR)	(1) Vertical jump	1 × 5 (SR) 2 × 5 (MR)	(1) High ankle hop	2 × 10 (MR)
(2) MB scoop toss	3 × 5	(2) DB quarter squat jump	1 × 5 (MR) 1 × 5 (MR)	(2) Power skip	2 × 4 each
(3) Deadlift	2 × 5 6 × 5,3,1,5,3,1	(3) Squat	2 × 5 4 × 5	(3) Bound	1 × 4 each (SR) 2 × 4 each (MR)
(4a) Pull-up (working sets: Wtd pull-up)	1 × 5 Work up to a 5RM then do 2 × 8 @ 80% of 5RM	(4a) RG bent-over row	1 × 5 4 × 5	(4) 40 yd build-ups	× 6
(4b) Glute-ham raise	4 × 10	(4b) Push-up on DBs	1 × 10% of ACFT HRP reps 4 × 50% of ACFT HRP reps		
(5a) Shoulder press	2 × 5 Work up to a 5RM then do 2 × 8 @ 80% of 5RM	(5a) SL RDL	3 × 8 each		
(5b) RG band pull-apart	4 × 15	(5b) Facepull	3 × 15		
(5c) Leg tuck	4 × 5-10	(5c) Roman side crunch	3 × 10 each		
Conditioning		**Conditioning**		**Conditioning**	
Backward sled drag (25 yds) + shuttle (25 yds)	× 6 with 1:3 W:R ratio	**15 min timed block:**	AMRAP	800 m repeats	× 5 at 5%-15% faster than 2-mile pace with 1:1 W:R ratio
		(a) 30 yd Sled push (in 15 yd increments)			
		(b) 30 yd DB farmer walk (in 15 yd increments)			

WEEK 2					
Day 1		**Day 2**		**Day 3**	
(1) Lateral bound	1 × 4 each (SR) 2 × 4 each (MR)	(1) Vertical jump	1 × 5 (SR) 2 × 5 (MR)	(1) High ankle hop	2 × 10 (MR)
(2) MB scoop toss	3 × 5	(2) DB quarter squat jump	*1 × 5 (MR)* 1 × 5 (MR)	(2) Power skip	2 × 4 each
(3) Deadlift	*2 × 5* 6 × 5,3,1,5,3,1	(3) Squat	*2 × 5* 4 × 5	(3) Bound	1 × 4 each (SR) 2 × 4 each (MR)
(4a) Pull-up (working sets: Wtd pull-up)	*1 × 5* Work up to a 5RM then do 2 × 8 @ 80% of 5RM	(4a) RG bent-over row	*1 × 5* 4 × 5	(4) 40 yd build-ups	× 6
(4b) Glute-ham raise	4 × 10	(4b) Push-up on DBs	*1 × 10% of ACFT HRP reps* 4 × 50% of ACFT HRP reps		
(5a) Shoulder press	*2 × 5* Work up to a 5RM then do 2 × 8 @ 80% of 5RM	(5a) SL RDL	3 × 8 each		
(5b) RG band pull-apart	4 × 15	(5b) Facepull	3 × 15		
(5c) Leg tuck	4 × 5-10	(5c) Roman side crunch	3 × 10 each		
Conditioning		**Conditioning**		**Conditioning**	
Backward sled drag (25 yds) + shuttle (25 yds)	× 6 with 1:3 W:R ratio	**15 min timed block:**	AMRAP	800 m repeats	× 5 at 5%-15% faster than 2-mile pace with 1:1 W:R ratio
		(a) 30 yd Sled push (in 15 yd increments)			
		(b) 30 yd DB farmer walk (in 15 yd increments)			

(continued)

Table 12.12   Three-Day Program, Phase 5 *(continued)*

WEEK 3					
Day 1		**Day 2**		**Day 3**	
(1) Lateral bound	1 × 4 each (SR) 2 × 4 each (MR)	(1) Vertical jump	1 × 5 (SR) 2 × 5 (MR)	(1) High ankle hop	2 × 10 (MR)
(2) MB scoop toss	3 × 5	(2) DB quarter squat jump	*1 × 5 (MR)* 1 × 5 (MR)	(2) Power skip	2 × 4 each
(3) Deadlift	*2 × 5* Work up to a 3RM	(3) Squat	*2 × 5* 4 × 5	(3) Bound	1 × 4 each (SR) 2 × 4 each (MR)
(4a) Pull-up (working sets: Wtd pull-up)	*1 × 5* Work up to a 3RM then do 2 × 6 @ 80% of 3RM	(4a) RG bent-over row	*1 × 5* 4 × 4	(4) 40 yd build-ups	× 6
(4b) Glute-ham raise	4 × 10	(4b) Push-up on DBs	*1 × 10% of ACFT HRP reps* 4 × 60% of ACFT HRP reps		
(5a) Shoulder press	*2 × 5* Work up to a 3RM then do 2 × 6 @ 80% of 3RM	(5a) SL RDL	3 × 8 each		
(5b) RG band pull-apart	4 × 15	(5b) Facepull	3 × 15		
(5c) Leg tuck	4 × 5-10	(5c) Roman side crunch	3 × 15 each		
Conditioning		**Conditioning**		**Conditioning**	
Backward sled drag (25 yds) + shuttle (25 yds)	× 6 with 1:3 W:R ratio	**15 min timed block:**	AMRAP	3-5 mile run	75%-85% MHR
		(a) 30 yd Sled push (in 15 yd increments)			
		(b) 30 yd DB farmer walk (in 15 yd increments)			

Three-Day Program, Phase 5

WEEK 4							
Day 1			**Day 2**			**Day 3**	
(1) Lateral bound	1 × 4 each (SR) 2 × 4 each (MR)		(1) Vertical jump	1 × 5 (SR) 2 × 5 (MR)		(1) High ankle hop	2 × 10 (MR)
(2) MB scoop toss	3 × 5		(2) DB quarter squat jump	1 × 5 (MR) 1 × 5 (MR)		(2) Power skip	2 × 4 each
(3) Deadlift	2 × 5 3 × 3		(3) Squat	2 × 5 3 × 5		(3) Bound	1 × 4 each (SR) 2 × 4 each (MR)
(4a) Pull-up	2 × 5 3 × 3		(4a) RG bent-over row	1 × 5 3 × 5		(4) 40 yd build-ups	× 6
(4b) Glute-ham raise	3 × 10		(4b) Push-up on DBs	1 × 10% of ACFT HRP reps 3 × 60% of ACFT HRP reps			
(5a) Shoulder press	2 × 5 3 × 3		(5a) SL RDL	3 × 8 each			
(5b) RG band pull-apart	4 × 15		(5b) Facepull	3 × 15			
(5c) Leg tuck	4 × 5-10		(5c) Roman side crunch	3 × 15 each			
Conditioning			**Conditioning**			**Conditioning**	
Backward sled drag (25 yds) + shuttle (25 yds)	× 6 with 1:3 W:R ratio		**15 min timed block:**	AMRAP		1 mile time trial	Rest 10 minutes
			(a) 30 yd Sled push (in 15 yd increments)			800 m repeats	× 2 at 5%-15% faster than 2-mile pace with 1:1 W:R ratio
			(b) 30 yd DB farmer walk (in 15 yd increments)				

Table 12.13   Three-Day Program, Phase 6

WEEK 1					
Day 1		**Day 2**		**Day 3**	
(1) Lateral bound	1 × 4 each (SR) 2 × 4 each (MR)	(1) High ankle hop	2 × 10 (MR)	(1) High ankle hop	1 × 10 (MR)
(2) 50 yd shuttle with alt foot plant	× 6	(2) Power skip	2 × 4 each	(2) Vertical jump	1 × 5 (SR)
(3) MB scoop toss	3 × 5	(3) Bound	1 × 4 each (SR) 2 × 4 each (MR)	(3) Power skip	2 × 4 each
(4a) Chin-up	2 × 5 4 × 8,8,6,6 1 × AMRAP (>5 reps)	(4) 40 yd build-ups	× 6	(4) ACFT practice	90% of previous ACFT results
(4b) RFE DB SA split squat	1 × 5 each 4 × 10 each				
(5a) Incline bench press	2 × 5 4 × 8,8,6,6				
(5b) RDL	1 × 5 3 × 5 1 × 10				
(6a) Leg tuck	4 × 5-20				
(6b) Facepull	4 × 15				
Conditioning		**Conditioning**		**Conditioning**	
8 rounds for time:		400 m repeats	× 9 at 5%-15% faster than 1-mile pace with 1:1 W:R ratio	None	
(a) Fan bike	15 calories				
(b) Hand release push-up	× 10				

WEEK 2					
Day 1		**Day 2**		**Day 3**	
(1) Lateral bound	1 × 4 each (SR) 2 × 4 each (MR)	(1) High ankle hop	2 × 10 (MR)	(1) High ankle hop	1 × 10 (MR)
(2) 50 yd shuttle with alt foot plant	× 6	(2) Power skip	2 × 4 each	(2) Vertical jump	1 × 5 (SR)
(3) MB scoop toss	3 × 5	(3) Bound	1 × 4 each (SR) 2 × 4 each (MR)	(3) Power skip	2 × 4 each
(4a) Chin-up	2 × 5 4 × 8,8,6,6 1 × AMRAP (>5 reps)	(4) 40 yd build-ups	× 6	(4) ACFT practice	100% of previous ACFT results
(4b) RFE DB SA split squat	1 × 5 each 4 × 10 each				
(5a) Incline bench press	2 × 5 4 × 8,8,6,6				
(5b) RDL	1 × 5 3 × 5 1 × 10				
(6a) Leg tuck	4 × 5-20				
(6b) Facepull	4 × 15				
Conditioning		**Conditioning**		**Conditioning**	
8 rounds for time:		400 m repeats	× 9 at 5%-15% faster than 1-mile pace with 1:1 W:R ratio	None	
(a) Fan bike	15 calories				
(b) Hand release push-up	× 10				

(continued)

Table 12.13   Three-Day Program, Phase 6 *(continued)*

WEEK 3					
Day 1		**Day 2**		**Day 3**	
(1) Lateral bound	1 × 4 each (SR) 2 × 4 each (MR)	(1) High ankle hop	2 × 10 (MR)	(1) High ankle hop	1 × 10 (MR)
(2) 50 yd shuttle with alt foot plant	× 6	(2) Power skip	2 × 4 each	(2) Vertical jump	1 × 5 (SR)
(3) MB scoop toss	3 × 5	(3) Bound	1 × 4 each (SR) 2 × 4 each (MR)	(3) Power skip	2 × 4 each
(4a) Chin-up	2 × 5 3 × 5	(4) 40 yd build-ups	× 6	(4) ACFT practice	All-out
(4b) RFE DB SA split squat	1 × 5 each 3 × 10 each				
(5a) Incline bench press	2 × 5 3 × 5				
(5b) RDL	1 × 5 3 × 5				
(6a) Leg tuck	4 × 5-20				
(6b) Facepull	4 × 15				
Conditioning		**Conditioning**		**Conditioning**	
8 rounds for time:		400 m repeats	× 9 at 5%-15% faster than 1-mile pace with 1:1 W:R ratio	None	
(a) Fan bike	15 calories				
(b) Hand release push-up	× 10				

WEEK 4					
Day 1		**Day 2**		**Day 3**	
(1) Lateral bound	1 × 4 each (SR) 1 × 4 each (MR)	(1) High ankle hop	2 × 10 (MR)	(1) High ankle hop	1 × 10 (MR)
(2) 50 yd shuttle with alt foot plant	× 4	(2) Power skip	2 × 4 each	(2) Vertical jump	1 × 5 (SR)
(3) MB scoop toss	3 × 5			(3) Power skip	2 × 4 each
(4a) Chin-up	2 × 5 3 × 5			(4) ACFT practice	80% of last week's ACFT results
(4b) RFE DB SA split squat	1 × 5 each 3 × 6 each				
(5a) Incline bench press	2 × 5 3 × 5				
(5b) RDL	1 × 5 3 × 5				
(6a) Leg tuck	2 × 5-20				
(6b) Facepull	2 × 15				
Conditioning		**Conditioning**		**Conditioning**	
6 rounds for time:		3-5 mile walk	No added weight	None	
(a) Fan bike	15 calories				
(b) Hand release push-up	× 10				

Table 12.14   Four-Day Program, Phase 1

WEEK 1						
Day 1		**Day 2**		**Day 3**		**Day 4**
(1) Vertical jump	2 × 5 (SR)	(1) High ankle hop	2 × 10 (MR)	(1) Vertical jump	2 × 5 (SR)	
(2a) DB walking lunge	1 × 8 each 3 × 12 each	(2) Power skip	2 × 4 each	(2a) Deadlift	2 × 5	
(2b) Shoulder press	2 × 5 3 × 10	(3) 40 yd build-ups	× 4	(2b) Push-up	2 × 10	
(2c) Ab rollout	3 × 12			(3) **EMOM circuit:**	15 min	
(3a) Pull-up	2 × 5 3 × 10			(a) Deadlift	× 2 @ 74% of ACFT MDL weight	
(3b) SB leg curl	3 × 12			(b) Push-up	15% of ACFT HRP reps	
(3c) Front plank	3 × 30 sec			(4a) Inverted row	3 × 12	
				(4b) Reverse crunch	3 × 12	
				(5a) Facepull	3 × 12	
				(5b) Side bend	3 × 12 each	
Conditioning		**Conditioning**		**Conditioning**		**Conditioning**
100 yd shuttle (in 25 yd increments)	× 6 with 2:30 rest	3-5 mile run	70%-80% MHR	None		5-6 mile ruck
WEEK 2						
Day 1		**Day 2**		**Day 3**		**Day 4**
(1) Vertical jump	2 × 5 (SR)	(1) High ankle hop	2 × 10 (MR)	(1) Vertical jump	2 × 5 (SR)	
(2a) DB walking lunge	1 × 8 each 3 × 12 each	(2) Power skip	2 × 4 each	(2a) Deadlift	2 × 5	
(2b) Shoulder press	2 × 5 3 × 10	(3) 40 yd build-ups	× 4	(2b) Push-up	2 × 10	
(2c) Ab rollout	3 × 12			(3) **EMOM circuit:**	20 min	
(3a) Pull-up	2 × 5 3 × 10			(a) Deadlift	× 2 @ 74% of ACFT MDL weight	
(3b) SB leg curl	3 × 12			(b) Push-up	15% of ACFT HRP reps	
(3c) Front plank	3 × 30 sec			(4a) Inverted row	3 × 12	
				(4b) Reverse crunch	3 × 12	
				(5a) Facepull	3 × 12	
				(5b) Side bend	3 × 12 each	
Conditioning		**Conditioning**		**Conditioning**		**Conditioning**
100 yd shuttle (in 25 yd increments)	× 6 with 2:30 rest	3-5 mile run	70%-80% MHR	None		5-6 mile ruck

In the Day 4 conditioning rows, the "70%-80% MHR" value appears in the second Day 4 column for both weeks.

WEEK 3						
Day 1		**Day 2**		**Day 3**		**Day 4**
(1) Vertical jump	2 × 5 (SR) 1 × 5 (MR)	(1) High ankle hop	2 × 10 (MR)	(1) Vertical jump	2 × 5 (SR)	
(2a) DB walking lunge	*1 × 8 each* 4 × 12 each	(2) Power skip	2 × 4 each	(2a) Deadlift	2 × 5	
(2b) Shoulder press	*2 × 5* 4 × 10	(3) 40 yd build-ups	× 4	(2b) Push-up	2 × 10	
(2c) Ab rollout	4 × 12			(3) **EMOM circuit:**	25 min	
(3a) Pull-up	*2 × 5* 4 × 10			(a) Deadlift	× 2 @ 74% of ACFT MDL weight	
(3b) SB leg curl	4 × 12			(b) Push-up	15% of ACFT HRP reps	
(3c) Front plank	4 × 30 sec			(4a) Inverted row	4 × 12	
				(4b) Reverse crunch	4 × 15	
				(5a) Facepull	4 × 12	
				(5b) Side bend	4 × 12 each	
Conditioning		**Conditioning**		**Conditioning**		**Conditioning**
100 yd shuttle (in 25 yd increments)	× 6 with 2:30 rest	3-5 mile run	70%-80% MHR	None		5-6 mile ruck	70%-80% MHR

WEEK 4						
Day 1		**Day 2**		**Day 3**		**Day 4**
(1) Vertical jump	2 × 5 (SR) 1 × 5 (MR)	(1) High ankle hop	2 × 10 (MR)	(1) Vertical jump	2 × 5 (SR)	
(2a) DB walking lunge	*1 × 8 each* 3 × 12 each	(2) Power skip	2 × 4 each	(2a) Deadlift	2 × 5	
(2b) Shoulder press	*2 × 5* 3 × 10	(3) 40 yd build-ups	× 4	(2b) Push-up	2 × 10	
(2c) Ab rollout	3 × 12			(3) **EMOM circuit:**	25 min	
(3a) Pull-up	*2 × 5* 3 × 10			(a) Deadlift	× 2 @ 74% of ACFT MDL weight	
(3b) SB leg curl	3 × 12			(b) Push-up	15% of ACFT HRP reps	
(3c) Front plank	3 × 30 sec			(4a) Inverted row	3 × 12	
				(4b) Reverse crunch	3 × 12	
				(5a) Facepull	3 × 12	
				(5b) Side bend	3 × 12 each	
Conditioning		**Conditioning**		**Conditioning**		**Conditioning**
100 yd shuttle (in 25 yd increments)	× 6 with 2:30 rest	3-5 mile run	70%-80% MHR	None		5-6 mile ruck	70%-80% MHR

Table 12.15   Four-Day Program, Phase 2

WEEK 1							
Day 1		**Day 2**		**Day 3**		**Day 4**	
(1) Vertical jump	1 × 5 (SR) 2 × 5 (MR)	(1a) Chin-up	2 × 5 4 × 8	(1) High ankle hop	2 × 10 (MR)	(1a) Deadbug arm only	2 × 5 each
(2) MB scoop toss	3 × 5	(1b) Shoulder press	2 × 5 4 × 8	(2) Power skip	2 × 4 each	(1b) Deadbug leg only	2 × 5 each
(3) Deadlift	2 × 5 4 × 5	(2a) DB bent-over row	1 × 5 3 × 15	(3) 40 yd build-ups	× 6	(2) Vertical jump	2 × 5 (SR) 1 × 5 (MR)
(4a) DB forward lunge	1 × 10 each 3 × 15 each	(2b) SA DB incline bench	1 × 5 each 3 × 15 each			(3a) RDL	2 × 5 4 × 5 (ECC3)
(4b) Lying trunk twist	3 × 8 each	(3a) DB biceps curl	3 × 15			(3b) Facepull	4 × 15
(5a) SB leg curl	3 × 15	(3b) Band pullapart	3 × 15			(4) **EMOM circuit:**	20 min
(5b) Ab rollout	3 × 15	(3c) Wtd plank	3 × 30 sec			(a) Pull-up	× 2
(5c) Triceps pushdown	3 × 12-15					(b) Push-up	× 4
						(c) Sit-up	× 4
						(d) Squat	× 4
Conditioning		**Conditioning**		**Conditioning**		**Conditioning**	
150 yd shuttle (in 25 yd increments)	× 6 with 2:30 rest	None		3-5 mile run	75%-85% MHR	Fan bike	4 × 30 sec with 4 min rest
WEEK 2							
Day 1		**Day 2**		**Day 3**		**Day 4**	
(1) Vertical jump	1 × 5 (SR) 2 × 5 (MR)	(1a) Chin-up	2 × 5 4 × 8	(1) High ankle hop	2 × 10 (MR)	(1a) Deadbug arm only	2 × 6 each
(2) MB scoop toss	3 × 5	(1b) Shoulder press	2 × 5 4 × 8	(2) Power skip	2 × 4 each	(1b) Deadbug leg only	2 × 6 each
(3) Deadlift	2 × 5 5 × 5	(2a) DB bent-over row	1 × 5 3 × 15	(3) 40 yd build-ups	× 6	(2) Vertical jump	1 × 5 (SR) 2 × 5 (MR)
(4a) DB forward lunge	1 × 10 each 3 × 15 each	(2b) SA DB incline bench	1 × 5 each 3 × 15 each			(3a) RDL	2 × 5 4 × 5 (ECC3)
(4b) Lying trunk twist	3 × 8 each	(3a) DB biceps curl	3 × 15			(3b) Facepull	4 × 15
(5a) SB leg curl	3 × 15	(3b) Band pullapart	3 × 15			(4) **EMOM circuit:**	20 min
(5b) Ab rollout	3 × 15	(3c) Wtd plank	3 × 30 sec			(a) Pull-up	× 2
(5c) Triceps pushdown	3 × 12-15					(b) Push-up	× 4
						(c) Sit-up	× 4
						(d) Squat	× 4
Conditioning		**Conditioning**		**Conditioning**		**Conditioning**	
150 yd shuttle (in 25 yd increments)	× 6 with 2:30 rest	None		5-6 mile ruck	75%-85% MHR	Fan bike	4 × 30 sec with 4 min rest

WEEK 3							
Day 1		**Day 2**		**Day 3**		**Day 4**	
(1) Vertical jump	1 × 5 (SR) 2 × 5 (MR)	(1a) Chin-up	2 × 5 4 × 8	(1) High ankle hop	2 × 10 (MR)	(1a) Deadbug arm only	2 × 8 each
(2) MB scoop toss	3 × 5	(1b) Shoulder press	2 × 5 4 × 8	(2) Power skip	2 × 4 each	(1b) Deadbug leg only	2 × 8 each
(3) Deadlift	2 × 5 5 × 5	(2a) DB bent-over row	1 × 5 3 × 15	(3) 40 yd build-ups	× 6	(2) Vertical jump	1 × 5 (SR) 2 × 5 (MR)
(4a) DB forward lunge	1 × 10 each 3 × 15 each	(2b) SA DB incline bench	1 × 5 each 3 × 15 each			(3a) RDL	2 × 5 4 × 5 (ECC3)
(4b) Lying trunk twist	4 × 8 each	(3a) DB biceps curl	3 × 15			(3b) Facepull	4 × 15
(5a) SB leg curl	3 × 15	(3b) Band pullapart	3 × 15			(4) **EMOM circuit:**	20 min
(5b) Ab rollout	3 × 15	(3c) Wtd plank	3 × 30 sec			(a) Pull-up	× 3
(5c) Triceps pushdown	3 × 12-15					(b) Push-up	× 5
						(c) Sit-up	× 5
						(d) Squat	× 7
Conditioning		**Conditioning**		**Conditioning**		**Conditioning**	
150 yd shuttle (in 25 yd increments)	× 6 with 2:30 rest	None		3-5 mile run	75%-85% MHR	Fan bike	4 × 30 sec with 3 min rest

WEEK 4							
Day 1		**Day 2**		**Day 3**		**Day 4**	
(1) Vertical jump	1 × 5 (SR) 2 × 5 (MR)	(1a) Chin-up	2 × 5 3 × 8	(1) High ankle hop	2 × 10 (MR)	(1a) Deadbug arm only	2 × 8 each
(2) MB scoop toss	3 × 5	(1b) Shoulder press	2 × 5 3 × 8	(2) Power skip	2 × 4 each	(1b) Deadbug leg only	2 × 8 each
(3) Deadlift	2 × 5 4 × 5	(2a) DB bent-over row	1 × 5 3 × 15	(3) 40 yd build-ups	× 6	(2) Vertical jump	1 × 5 (SR) 2 × 5 (MR)
(4a) DB forward lunge	1 × 10 each 3 × 15 each	(2b) SA DB incline bench	1 × 5 each 3 × 15 each			(3a) RDL	2 × 5 3 × 8
(4b) Lying trunk twist	4 × 8 each	(3a) DB biceps curl	3 × 15			(3b) Facepull	4 × 15
(5a) SB leg curl	3 × 15	(3b) Band pullapart	3 × 15			(4) **EMOM circuit:**	20 min
(5b) Ab rollout	3 × 15	(3c) Wtd plank	3 × 30 sec			(a) Pull-up	× 3
(5c) Triceps pushdown	3 × 12-15					(b) Push-up	× 5
						(c) Sit-up	× 5
						(d) Squat	× 7
Conditioning		**Conditioning**		**Conditioning**		**Conditioning**	
150 yd shuttle (in 25 yd increments)	× 6 with 2:30 rest	None		5-6 mile ruck	75%-85% MHR	Fan bike	4 × 30 sec with 3 min rest

Four-Day Program, Phase 3

Table 12.16   Four-Day Program, Phase 3

WEEK 1							
Day 1		**Day 2**		**Day 3**		**Day 4**	
(1) Lateral bound	3 × 4 each (SR)	(1) High ankle hop	2 × 10 (MR)	(1) Vertical jump	3 × 5 (SR)	(1) Deadbug	2 × 8 each
(2) Squat	2 × 5 4 × 5	(2) Power skip	2 × 4 each	(2) MB scoop toss	3 × 5	(2a) Broad jump	3 × 3 (SR)
(3a) Bent-over row	1 × 5 4 × 5	(3) 40 yd build-ups	× 6	(3) Deadlift	2 × 5 4 × 5	(2b) Chin-up	1 × 5 4 × 5
(3b) DB incline press	1 × 5 4 × 10			(4a) Alt DB prone row	1 × 5 each 4 × 10 each	(3a) Shoulder press	2 × 5 4 × 5
(4a) SA/SL DB RDL	3 × 10 each			(4b) Glute-ham raise	4 × 10	(3b) DB reverse lunge	1 × 5 each 4 × 10 each
(4b) Rear deltoid raise	3 × 10			(4c) Sit-up	4 × 20	(4a) RDL	1 × 5 4 × 5 (ISO3)
(4c) Ab rollout	3 × 10			(5a) Bench press	2 × 5 4 × 5	(4b) Band pullapart	4 × 15
				(5b) Facepull	4 × 15	(4c) Stir the pot	4 × 3 each with 4 sec circles
				(5c) Pallof press	4 × 5 each side (ECC5)		
Conditioning		**Conditioning**		**Conditioning**		**Conditioning**	
Rower time trial	500 m × 3 with 5 min rest	1 mile repeats	× 3 at 2-mile pace with 1:1 W:R ratio	**15 min timed block:**	AMRAP	Fan bike	4 × 30 sec with 3 min rest
				(a) 30 yd Sled push (in 15 yd increments)			
				(b) 30 yd DB farmer walk (in 15 yd increments)			

WEEK 2							
Day 1		**Day 2**		**Day 3**		**Day 4**	
(1) Lateral bound	3 × 4 each (SR)	(1) High ankle hop	2 × 10 (MR)	(1) Vertical jump	3 × 5 (SR)	(1) Deadbug	2 × 8 each
(2) Squat	*2 × 5* 4 × 5	(2) Power skip	2 × 4 each	(2) MB scoop toss	3 × 5	(2a) Broad jump	3 × 3 (SR)
(3a) Bent-over row	*1 × 5* 4 × 5	(3) 40 yd build-ups	× 6	(3) Deadlift	*2 × 5* 4 × 5	(2b) Chin-up	*1 × 5* 4 × 5
(3b) DB incline press	*1 × 5* 4 × 10			(4a) Alt DB prone row	*1 × 5* each 4 × 10 each	(3a) Shoulder press	*2 × 5* 4 × 5
(4a) SA/SL DB RDL	3 × 10 each			(4b) Glute-ham raise	4 × 10	(3b) DB reverse lunge	*1 × 5 each* 4 × 10 each
(4b) Rear deltoid raise	3 × 10			(4c) Sit-up	4 × 20	(4a) RDL	*1 × 5* 4 × 5 (ISO3)
(4c) Ab rollout	3 × 10			(5a) Bench press	*2 × 5* 4 × 5	(4b) Band pullapart	4 × 15
				(5b) Facepull	4 × 15	(4c) Stir the pot	4 × 5 each with 4 sec circles
				(5c) Pallof press	4 × 5 each side (ECC5)		
Conditioning		**Conditioning**		**Conditioning**		**Conditioning**	
Rower time trial	500 m × 3 with 5 min rest	1 mile repeats	× 3 at 2-mile pace with 1:1 W:R ratio	**15 min timed block:**	AMRAP	Fan bike	5 × 30 sec with 3 min rest
				(a) 30 yd Sled push (in 15 yd increments)			
				(b) 30 yd DB farmer walk (in 15 yd increments)			

(continued)

Four-Day Program, Phase 3

Table 12.16   Four-Day Program, Phase 3 *(continued)*

WEEK 3							
Day 1		**Day 2**		**Day 3**		**Day 4**	
(1) Lateral bound	3 × 4 each (SR)	(1) High ankle hop	2 × 10 (MR)	(1) Vertical jump	3 × 5 (SR)	(1) Deadbug	3 × 8 each
(2) Squat	2 × 5 4 × 3	(2) Power skip	2 × 4 each	(2) MB scoop toss	3 × 5	(2a) Broad jump	3 × 3 (SR)
(3a) Bent-over row	1 × 5 4 × 4	(3) 40 yd build-ups	× 6	(3) Deadlift	2 × 5 4 × 3	(2b) Chin-up	1 × 5 4 × 3
(3b) DB incline press	1 × 5 4 × 8			(4a) Alt DB prone row	1 × 5 each 4 × 8 each	(3a) Shoulder press	2 × 5 4 × 3
(4a) SA/SL DB RDL	3 × 8 each			(4b) Glute-ham raise	4 × 10	(3b) DB reverse lunge	1 × 5 each 4 × 8 each
(4b) Rear deltoid raise	3 × 10			(4c) Sit-up	4 × 25	(4a) RDL	1 × 5 4 × 5 (ISO3)
(4c) Ab rollout	3 × 10			(5a) Bench press	2 × 5 4 × 3	(4b) Band pullapart	4 × 15
				(5b) Facepull	4 × 15	(4c) Stir the pot	4 × 5 each with 4 sec circles
				(5c) Pallof press	4 × 10 each side (ECC3)		
Conditioning		**Conditioning**		**Conditioning**		**Conditioning**	
Rower time trial	500 m × 3 with 5 min rest	1 mile repeats	× 3 at 2-mile pace with 1:1 W:R ratio	**15 min timed block:**	AMRAP	Fan bike	5 × 30 sec with 3 min rest
				(a) 30 yd Sled push (in 15 yd increments)			
				(b) 30 yd DB farmer walk (in 15 yd increments)			

WEEK 4							
Day 1		**Day 2**		**Day 3**		**Day 4**	
(1) Lateral bound	3 × 4 each (SR)	(1) High ankle hop	2 × 10 (MR)	(1) Vertical jump	3 × 5 (SR)	(1) Deadbug	3 × 8 each
(2) Squat	2 × 5 4 × 3	(2) Power skip	2 × 4 each	(2) MB scoop toss	2 × 5	(2a) Broad jump	3 × 3 (SR)
(3a) Bent-over row	1 × 5 3 × 4	(3) 40 yd build-ups	× 6	(3) Deadlift	2 × 5 4 × 3	(2b) Chin-up	1 × 5 4 × 3
(3b) DB incline press	1 × 5 4 × 8			(4a) Alt DB prone row	1 × 5 each 3 × 8 each	(3a) Shoulder press	2 × 5 4 × 3
(4a) SA/SL DB RDL	3 × 8 each			(4b) Glute-ham raise	3 × 10	(3b) DB reverse lunge	1 × 5 each 3 × 8 each
(4b) Rear deltoid raise	3 × 10			(4c) Sit-up	3 × 25	(4a) RDL	1 × 5 3 × 5
(4c) Ab rollout	3 × 10			(5a) Bench press	2 × 5 3 × 3	(4b) Band pullapart	3 × 15
				(5b) Facepull	3 × 15	(4c) Stir the pot	4 × 5 each with 4 sec circles
				(5c) Pallof press	4 × 10 each side (ECC3)		
Conditioning		**Conditioning**		**Conditioning**		**Conditioning**	
Rower time trial	500 m × 3 with 5 min rest	1 mile repeats	× 3 at 2-mile pace with 1:1 W:R ratio	**15 min timed block:**	AMRAP	Fan bike	5 × 30 sec with 3 min rest
				(a) 30 yd Sled push (in 15 yd increments)			
				(b) 30 yd DB farmer walk (in 15 yd increments)			

Four-Day Program, Phase 4

Table 12.17   Four-Day Program, Phase 4

WEEK 1							
Day 1		**Day 2**		**Day 3**		**Day 4**	
(1) Lateral bound	1 × 4 each (SR) 2 × 4 each (MR)	(1) High ankle hop	2 × 10 (MR)	(1) Vertical jump	1 × 5 (SR) 2 × 5 (MR)	(1) Broad jump	1 × 3 (SR) 2 × 3 (MR)
(2) DB quarter squat jump	1 × 5 (SR) 2 × 5 (SR)	(2) Bound	2 × 4 each (SR)	(2) Tuck jump	2 × 5 (MR)	(2) Hang clean low pull	1 × 5 2 × 5
(3) Squat	2 × 5 4 × 5	(3) Power skip	2 × 4 each	(3a) Deadlift	2 × 5 4 × 5	(3) Pull-up	1 × 5 4 × 5
(4a) RG bent-over row	1 × 5 4 × 5	(4) 40 yd build-ups	× 6	(3b) MB scoop toss	4 × 5	(4a) Shoulder press	2 × 5 4 × 5
(4b) Wtd push-up	1 × 10 4 × 10			(4a) DB prone row	1 × 5 4 × 10	(4b) DB forward lunge	1 × 5 each 4 × 10 each
(5a) DB SL RDL	3 × 10 each			(4b) Poor man's glute-ham raise	4 × 5	(5a) RDL	1 × 5 4 × 5
(5b) Facepull	3 × 15			(5a) Bench press	2 × 5 4 × 5	(5b) Rear deltoid raise	3 × 10
(5c) Hanging knee raise	3 × 12			(5b) RG band pull-apart	4 × 15	(5c) Eccentric dragon flag	3 × 10
				(5c) Ab rollout	3 × 12		
Conditioning		**Conditioning**		**Conditioning**		**Conditioning**	
150 yd shuttle (in 25 yd increments)	× 5 with 1:30 rest	400 m repeats	× 9 at 5%-15% faster than 2-mile pace with 1:1 W:R ratio	Rower time trial	500 m × 3 with 1:3 W:R ratio	**8 rounds for time:**	
						(a) Fan bike	15 calories
						(b) Hand release push-up	× 10

Four-Day Program, Phase 4

WEEK 2							
Day 1		**Day 2**		**Day 3**		**Day 4**	
(1) Lateral bound	1 × 4 each (SR) 2 × 4 each (MR)	(1) High ankle hop	2 × 10 (MR)	(1) Vertical jump	1 × 5 (SR) 2 × 5 (MR)	(1) Broad jump	1 × 3 (SR) 2 × 3 (MR)
(2) DB quarter squat jump	1 × 5 (SR) 2 × 5 (SR)	(2) Bound	2 × 4 each (SR)	(2) Tuck jump	2 × 5 (MR)	(2) Hang clean low pull	1 × 5 3 × 5
(3) Squat	2 × 5 4 × 3	(3) Power skip	2 × 4 each	(3a) Deadlift	2 × 5 4 × 3	(3) Pull-up	1 × 5 4 × 3
(4a) RG bent-over row	1 × 5 4 × 5	(4) 40 yd build-ups	× 6	(3b) MB scoop toss	3 × 5	(4a) Shoulder press	2 × 5 4 × 3
(4b) Wtd push-up	1 × 10 4 × 8			(4a) DB prone row	1 × 5 4 × 8	(4b) DB forward lunge	1 × 5 each 4 × 8 each
(5a) DB SL RDL	3 × 8 each			(4b) Poor man's glute-ham raise	4 × 5	(5a) RDL	1 × 5 4 × 5
(5b) Facepull	3 × 15			(5a) Bench press	2 × 5 4 × 3	(5b) Rear deltoid raise	3 × 10
(5c) Hanging knee raise	3 × 15			(5b) RG band pull-apart	4 × 15	(5c) Eccentric dragon flag	3 × 10
				(5c) Ab rollout	3 × 12		
Conditioning		**Conditioning**		**Conditioning**		**Conditioning**	
150 yd shuttle (in 25 yd increments)	× 5 with 1:30 rest	400 m repeats	× 9 at 5%-15% faster than 2-mile pace with 1:1 W:R ratio	Rower time trial	500 m × 3 with 1:3 W:R ratio	**8 rounds for time:**	
						(a) Fan bike	15 calories
						(b) Hand release push-up	× 10

(continued)

Table 12.17   Four-Day Program, Phase 4 *(continued)*

WEEK 3							
Day 1		**Day 2**		**Day 3**		**Day 4**	
(1) Lateral bound	1 × 4 each (SR) 2 × 4 each (MR)	(1) High ankle hop	2 × 10 (MR)	(1) Vertical jump	1 × 5 (SR) 2 × 5 (MR)	(1) Broad jump	1 × 3 (SR) 2 × 3 (MR)
(2) DB quarter squat jump	1 × 5 (SR) 2 × 5 (SR)	(2) Bound	2 × 4 each (SR)	(2) Tuck jump	2 × 5 (MR)	(2) Hang clean low pull	1 × 5 3 × 5
(3) Squat	2 × 5 4 × 3,2,1,1	(3) Power skip	2 × 4 each	(3a) Deadlift	2 × 5 4 × 3	(3) Pull-up	1 × 5 4 × 3,2,2,2
(4a) RG bent-over row	1 × 5 4 × 4	(4) 40 yd build-ups	× 6	(3b) MB scoop toss	3 × 5	(4a) Shoulder press	2 × 5 4 × 3,2,2,2
(4b) Wtd push-up	1 × 10 4 × 8			(4a) DB prone row	1 × 5 4 × 8	(4b) DB forward lunge	1 × 5 each 4 × 8 each
(5a) DB SL RDL	3 × 8 each			(4b) Poor man's glute-ham raise	4 × 6	(5a) RDL	1 × 5 4 × 5
(5b) Facepull	3 × 15			(5a) Bench press	2 × 5 4 × 3,2,1,1	(5b) Rear deltoid raise	3 × 10
(5c) Hanging knee raise	3 × 15			(5b) RG band pull-apart	4 × 15	(5c) Eccentric dragon flag	3 × 10
				(5c) Ab rollout	3 × 15		
Conditioning		**Conditioning**		**Conditioning**		**Conditioning**	
150 yd shuttle (in 25 yd increments)	× 5 with 1:30 rest	3-5 mile run	75%-85% MHR	Rower time trial	500 m × 3 with 1:3 W:R ratio	**8 rounds for time:**	
						(a) Fan bike	15 calories
						(b) Hand release push-up	× 10

WEEK 4							
Day 1		**Day 2**		**Day 3**		**Day 4**	
(1) Lateral bound	1 × 4 each (SR) 2 × 4 each (MR)	(1) High ankle hop	2 × 10 (MR)	(1) Vertical jump	1 × 5 (SR) 2 × 5 (MR)	(1) Broad jump	1 × 3 (SR) 2 × 3 (MR)
(2) DB quarter squat jump	*1 × 5 (SR)* 2 × 5 (SR)	(2) Bound	2 × 4 each (SR)	(2) Tuck jump	2 × 5 (MR)	(2) Hang clean low pull	*1 × 5* 3 × 5
(3) Squat	*2 × 5* 3 × 3	(3) Power skip	2 × 4 each	(3a) Deadlift	*2 × 5* 4 × 3,2,1,1	(3) Pull-up	*1 × 5* 3 × 3
(4a) RG bent-over row	*1 × 5* 3 × 4	(4) 40 yd build-ups	× 6	(3b) MB scoop toss	2 × 4	(4a) Shoulder press	*2 × 5* 3 × 3
(4b) Wtd push-up	*1 × 10* 3 × 8			(4a) DB prone row	*1 × 5* 3 × 8	(4b) DB forward lunge	*1 × 5 each* 3 × 8 each
(5a) DB SL RDL	3 × 8 each			(4b) Poor man's glute-ham raise	3 × 5	(5a) RDL	*1 × 5* 3 × 5
(5b) Facepull	3 × 15			(5a) Bench press	*2 × 5* 3 × 3	(5b) Rear deltoid raise	3 × 10
(5c) Hanging knee raise	3 × 15			(5b) RG band pull-apart	4 × 15	(5c) Eccentric dragon flag	3 × 10
				(5c) Ab rollout	3 × 15		
Conditioning		**Conditioning**		**Conditioning**		**Conditioning**	
150 yd shuttle (in 25 yd increments)	× 5 with 1:30 rest	400 m repeats	× 9 at 5%-15% faster than 2-mile pace with 1:1 W:R ratio	Rower time trial	500 m × 3 with 1:3 W:R ratio	**8 rounds for time:**	
						(a) Fan bike	15 calories
						(b) Hand release push-up	× 10

Table 12.18   Four-Day Program, Phase 5

WEEK 1							
Day 1		**Day 2**		**Day 3**		**Day 4**	
(1) Lateral bound	1 × 4 each (SR) 2 × 4 each (MR)	(1) High ankle hop	2 × 10 (MR)	(1) Vertical jump	1 × 5 (SR) 2 × 5 (MR)	(1) Broad jump	1 × 3 (SR) 2 × 3 (MR)
(2) MB scoop toss	3 × 5	(2) Power skip	2 × 4 each	(2) DB quarter squat jump	1 × 5 (MR) 1 × 5 (MR)	(2) Hang clean low pull	2 × 5 3 × 5
(3) Deadlift	2 × 5 6 × 5,3,1,5,3,1	(3) Bound	1 × 4 each (SR) 2 × 4 each (MR)	(3) Squat	2 × 5 4 × 5	(3) Pull-up (working sets: Wtd pull-up)	1 × 5 Work up to a 5RM then do 2 × 8 @ 80% of 5RM
(4a) DB prone row	1 × 5 4 × 10	(4) 40 yd build-ups	× 6	(4a) RG bent-over row	1 × 5 4 × 5	(4a) Shoulder press	2 × 5 Work up to a 5RM then do 2 × 8 @ 80% of 5RM
(4b) Glute-ham raise	4 × 10			(4b) Push-up on DBs	1 × 10% of ACFT HRP reps 4 × 50% of ACFT HRP reps	(4b) Lateral squat	1 × 5 each 3 × 10 each
(5a) Bench press	2 × 5 Work up to a 5RM then do 2 × 8 @ 80% of 5RM			(5a) SL RDL	3 × 8 each	(5a) RDL	1 × 5 3 × 10
(5b) RG band pullapart	4 × 15			(5b) Facepull	3 × 15	(5b) Rear deltoid raise	3 × 10
(5c) Leg tuck	4 × 5-10			(5c) Roman side crunch	3 × 10 each	(5c) Landmine twist	3 × 6 each
Conditioning		**Conditioning**		**Conditioning**		**Conditioning**	
Backward sled drag (25 yds) + shuttle (25 yds)	× 6 with 1:3 W:R ratio	800 m repeats	× 5 at 5%-15% faster than 2-mile pace with 1:1 W:R ratio	**6 rounds for time:**		**15 min timed block:**	AMRAP
				(a) Rower	500 m	(a) 30 yd Sled push (in 15 yd increments)	
				(b) Hand release push-up	× 10	(b) 30 yd DB farmer walk (in 15 yd increments)	

Four-Day Program, Phase 5

WEEK 2							
Day 1		**Day 2**		**Day 3**		**Day 4**	
(1) Lateral bound	1 × 4 each (SR) 2 × 4 each (MR)	(1) High ankle hop	2 × 10 (MR)	(1) Vertical jump	1 × 5 (SR) 2 × 5 (MR)	(1) Broad jump	1 × 3 (SR) 2 × 3 (MR)
(2) MB scoop toss	3 × 5	(2) Power skip	2 × 4 each	(2) DB quarter squat jump	1 × 5 (MR) 1 × 5 (MR)	(2) Hang clean low pull	2 × 5 3 × 5
(3) Deadlift	2 × 5 6 × 5,3,1,5,3,1	(3) Bound	1 × 4 each (SR) 2 × 4 each (MR)	(3) Squat	2 × 5 4 × 5	(3) Pull-up (working sets: Wtd pull-up)	1 × 5 Work up to a 3RM then do 2 × 6 @ 80% of 3RM
(4a) DB prone row	1 × 5 4 × 10	(4) 40 yd build-ups	× 6	(4a) RG bent-over row	1 × 5 4 × 5	(4a) Shoulder press	2 × 5 Work up to a 3RM then do 2 × 6 @ 80% of 3RM
(4b) Glute-ham raise	4 × 10			(4b) Push-up on DBs	1 × 10% of ACFT HRP reps 4 × 50% of ACFT HRP reps	(4b) Lateral squat	1 × 5 each 3 × 10 each
(5a) Bench press	2 × 5 Work up to a 3RM then do 2 × 6 @ 80% of 3RM			(5a) SL RDL	3 × 8 each	(5a) RDL	1 × 5 3 × 10
(5b) RG band pullapart	4 × 15			(5b) Facepull	3 × 15	(5b) Rear deltoid raise	4 × 10
(5c) Leg tuck	4 × 5-10			(5c) Roman side crunch	3 × 10 each	(5c) Landmine twist	3 × 8 each
Conditioning		**Conditioning**		**Conditioning**		**Conditioning**	
Backward sled drag (25 yds) + shuttle (25 yds)	× 6 with 1:3 W:R ratio	800 m repeats	× 5 at 5%-15% faster than 2-mile pace with 1:1 W:R ratio	**6 rounds for time:**		**15 min timed block:**	AMRAP
				(a) Rower	500 m	(a) 30 yd Sled push (in 15 yd increments)	
				(b) Hand release push-up	× 10	(b) 30 yd DB farmer walk (in 15 yd increments)	

(continued)

Table 12.18   Four-Day Program, Phase 5 *(continued)*

WEEK 3							
Day 1		**Day 2**		**Day 3**		**Day 4**	
(1) Lateral bound	1 × 4 each (SR) 2 × 4 each (MR)	(1) High ankle hop	2 × 10 (MR)	(1) Vertical jump	1 × 5 (SR) 2 × 5 (MR)	(1) Broad jump	1 × 3 (SR) 2 × 3 (MR)
(2) MB scoop toss	3 × 5	(2) Power skip	2 × 4 each	(2) DB quarter squat jump	1 × 5 (MR) 1 × 5 (MR)	(2) Hang clean low pull	2 × 5 3 × 5
(3) Deadlift	2 × 5 Work up to a 3RM	(3) Bound	1 × 4 each (SR) 2 × 4 each (MR)	(3) Squat	2 × 5 4 × 5	(3) Pull-up (working sets: Wtd pull-up)	1 × 5 Work up to a 3RM then do 2 × 6 @ 80% of 3RM
(4a) DB prone row	1 × 5 4 × 10	(4) 40 yd build-ups	× 6	(4a) RG bent-over row	1 × 5 4 × 4	(4a) Shoulder press	2 × 5 Work up to a 3RM then do 2 × 6 @ 80% of 3RM
(4b) Glute-ham raise	4 × 10			(4b) Push-up on DBs	1 × 10% of ACFT HRP reps 4 × 60% of ACFT HRP reps	(4b) Lateral squat	1 × 5 each 3 × 8 each
(5a) Bench press	2 × 5 Work up to a 1RM then do 2 × 4 @ 80% 1RM			(5a) SL RDL	3 × 8 each	(5a) RDL	1 × 5 3 × 8
(5b) RG band pullapart	4 × 10			(5b) Facepull	3 × 15	(5b) Rear deltoid raise	4 × 10
(5c) Leg tuck	4 × 5-15			(5c) Roman side crunch	3 × 15 each	(5c) Landmine twist	3 × 10 each
Conditioning		**Conditioning**		**Conditioning**		**Conditioning**	
Backward sled drag (25 yds) + shuttle (25 yds)	× 6 with 1:3 W:R ratio	3-5 mile run	75%-85% MHR	**6 rounds for time:**		**15 min timed block:**	AMRAP
				(a) Rower	500 m	(a) 30 yd Sled push (in 15 yd increments)	
				(b) Hand release push-up	× 10	(b) 30 yd DB farmer walk (in 15 yd increments)	

WEEK 4							
Day 1		**Day 2**		**Day 3**		**Day 4**	
(1) Lateral bound	1 × 4 each (SR) 2 × 4 each (MR)	(1) High ankle hop	2 × 10 (MR)	(1) Vertical jump	1 × 5 (SR) 2 × 5 (MR)	(1) Broad jump	1 × 3 (SR) 2 × 3 (MR)
(2) MB scoop toss	3 × 5	(2) Power skip	2 × 4 each	(2) DB quarter squat jump	1 × 5 (MR) 1 × 5 (MR)	(2) Hang clean low pull	2 × 5 3 × 5
(3) Deadlift	2 × 5 3 × 3	(3) Bound	1 × 4 each (SR) 2 × 4 each (MR)	(3) Squat	2 × 5 3 × 5	(3) Pull-up	1 × 5 3 × 3
(4a) DB prone row	1 × 5 3 × 10	(4) 40 yd build-ups	× 6	(4a) RG bent-over row	1 × 5 4 × 4	(4a) Shoulder press	2 × 5 3 × 3
(4b) Glute-ham raise	3 × 10			(4b) Push-up on DBs	1 × 10% of ACFT HRP reps 3 × 60% of ACFT HRP reps	(4b) Lateral squat	1 × 5 each 3 × 8 each
(5a) Bench press	2 × 5 3 × 5			(5a) SL RDL	3 × 8 each	(5a) RDL	1 × 5 3 × 8
(5b) RG band pullapart	4 × 10			(5b) Facepull	3 × 15	(5b) Rear deltoid raise	4 × 10
(5c) Leg tuck	4 × 5-15			(5c) Roman side crunch	3 × 15 each	(5c) Landmine twist	3 × 10 each
Conditioning		**Conditioning**		**Conditioning**		**Conditioning**	
Backward sled drag (25 yds) + shuttle (25 yds)	× 6 with 1:3 W:R ratio	1 mile time trial	Rest 10 minutes	**6 rounds for time:**		**15 min timed block:**	AMRAP
		800 m repeats	× 2 at 5%-15% faster than 2-mile pace with 1:1 W:R ratio	(a) Rower	500 m	(a) 30 yd Sled push (in 15 yd increments)	
				(b) Hand release push-up	× 10	(b) 30 yd DB farmer walk (in 15 yd increments)	

Table 12.19   Four-Day Program, Phase 6

WEEK 1							
Day 1		**Day 2**		**Day 3**		**Day 4**	
(1) High ankle hop	2 × 10 (MR)	(1) Broad jump	1 × 3 (SR) 2 × 3 (MR)	(1) Vertical jump	1 × 5 (SR) 2 × 5 (MR)	(1) High ankle hop	1 × 10 (MR)
(2) Power skip	2 × 4 each	(2) Lateral bound	1 × 4 each (SR) 2 × 4 each (MR)	(2) 50 yd shuttle with alt foot plant	× 6	(2) Vertical jump	1 × 5 (SR)
(3) Bound	1 × 4 each (SR) 2 × 4 each (MR)	(3) MB scoop toss	3 × 5	(3) Hang clean low pull	2 × 5 4 × 3	(3) Power skip	2 × 4 each
(4) 40 yd build-ups	× 6	(4a) Chin-up	2 × 5 4 × 8,8,6,6 1 × AMRAP (>5 reps)	(4a) Inverted row	1 × 5 4 × 10	(4) ACFT practice	90% of previous ACFT results
		(4b) Lateral squat	1 × 5 each 4 × 5 each	(4b) Body saw	4 × 10		
		(5a) Incline bench press	2 × 5 4 × 8,8,6,6	(5a) SA DB shoulder press	1 × 5 each 4 × 10 each		
		(5b) SB leg curl	4 × 15	(5b) RFE DB SA split squat	1 × 5 each 4 × 10 each		
		(6a) Leg tuck	4 × 5-20	(6a) RDL	1 × 5 3 × 5 1 × 10		
		(6b) Facepull	4 × 15	(6b) RG band pull-apart	4 × 15		
Conditioning		**Conditioning**		**Conditioning**		**Conditioning**	
400 m repeats	× 9 at 5%-15% faster than 1-mile pace with 1:1 W:R ratio	**8 rounds for time:**		None		None	
		(a) Fan bike	15 calories				
		(b) Hand release push-up	× 10				

WEEK 2							
Day 1		**Day 2**		**Day 3**		**Day 4**	
(1) High ankle hop	2 × 10 (MR)	(1) Broad jump	1 × 3 (SR) 2 × 3 (MR)	(1) Vertical jump	1 × 5 (SR) 2 × 5 (MR)	(1) High ankle hop	1 × 10 (MR)
(2) Power skip	2 × 4 each	(2) Lateral bound	1 × 4 each (SR) 2 × 4 each (MR)	(2) 50 yd shuttle with alt foot plant	× 6	(2) Vertical jump	1 × 5 (SR)
(3) Bound	1 × 4 each (SR) 2 × 4 each (MR)	(3) MB scoop toss	3 × 5	(3) Hang clean low pull	2 × 5 4 × 3	(3) Power skip	2 × 4 each
(4) 40 yd build-ups	× 6	(4a) Chin-up	2 × 5 4 × 8,8,6,6 1 × AMRAP (>5 reps)	(4a) Inverted row	1 × 5 4 × 10	(4) ACFT practice	100% of previous ACFT results
		(4b) Lateral squat	1 × 5 each 4 × 5 each	(4b) Body saw	4 × 10		
		(5a) Incline bench press	2 × 5 4 × 8,8,6,6	(5a) SA DB shoulder press	1 × 5 each 4 × 10 each		
		(5b) SB leg curl	4 × 15	(5b) RFE DB SA split squat	1 × 5 each 4 × 10 each		
		(6a) Leg tuck	4 × 5-20	(6a) RDL	1 × 5 3 × 5 1 × 10		
		(6b) Facepull	3 × 15	(6b) RG band pull-apart	4 × 15		
Conditioning		**Conditioning**		**Conditioning**		**Conditioning**	
3-5 mile run	75%-85% MHR	**8 rounds for time:**		None		None	
		(a) Fan bike	15 calories				
		(b) Hand release push-up	× 10				

(continued)

Table 12.19   **Four-Day Program, Phase 6** *(continued)*

WEEK 3							
Day 1		**Day 2**		**Day 3**		**Day 4**	
(1) High ankle hop	2 × 10 (MR)	(1) Broad jump	1 × 3 (SR) 2 × 3 (MR)	(1) Vertical jump	1 × 5 (SR) 2 × 5 (MR)	(1) High ankle hop	1 × 10 (MR)
(2) Power skip	2 × 4 each	(2) Lateral bound	1 × 4 each (SR) 2 × 4 each (MR)	(2) 50 yd shuttle with alt foot plant	× 6	(2) Vertical jump	1 × 5 (SR)
(3) Bound	1 × 4 each (SR) 2 × 4 each (MR)	(3) MB scoop toss	3 × 5	(3) Hang clean low pull	2 × 5 3 × 3	(3) Power skip	2 × 4 each
(4) 40 yd build-ups	× 6	(4a) Chin-up	2 × 5 3 × 5	(4a) Inverted row	1 × 5 3 × 10	(4) ACFT practice	All-out
		(4b) Lateral squat	1 × 5 each 3 × 5 each	(4b) Body saw	4 × 10		
		(5a) Incline bench press	2 × 5 3 × 5	(5a) SA DB shoulder press	1 × 5 each 3 × 10 each		
		(5b) SB leg curl	4 × 10	(5b) RFE DB SA split squat	1 × 5 each 3 × 10 each		
		(6a) Leg tuck	4 × 5-20	(6a) RDL	1 × 5 3 × 5		
		(6b) Facepull	3 × 15	(6b) RG band pull-apart	4 × 15		
Conditioning		**Conditioning**		**Conditioning**		**Conditioning**	
400 m repeats	× 9 at 5%-15% faster than 1-mile pace with 1:1 W:R ratio	**8 rounds for time:**		None		None	
		(a) Fan bike	15 calories				
		(b) Hand release push-up	× 10				

Four-Day Program, Phase 6

WEEK 4							
Day 1		**Day 2**		**Day 3**		**Day 4**	
(1) High ankle hop	2 × 10 (MR)	(1) Broad jump	1 × 3 (SR) 2 × 3 (MR)	(1) Vertical jump	1 × 5 (SR) 2 × 5 (MR)	(1) High ankle hop	1 × 10 (MR)
(2) Power skip	2 × 4 each	(2) Lateral bound	1 × 4 each (SR) 1 × 4 each (MR)	(2) 50 yd shuttle with alt foot plant	× 4	(2) Vertical jump	1 × 5 (SR)
(3) 40 yd build-ups	× 4	(3) MB scoop toss	3 × 5	(3) Hang clean low pull	2 × 5 3 × 3	(3) Power skip	2 × 4 each
		(4a) Chin-up	2 × 5 3 × 5	(4a) Inverted row	1 × 5 3 × 10	(4) ACFT practice	80% of last week's ACFT results
		(4b) Lateral squat	1 × 5 each 2 × 5 each	(4b) Body saw	3 × 10		
		(5a) Incline bench press	2 × 5 3 × 5	(5a) SA DB shoulder press	1 × 5 each 3 × 6 each		
		(5b) SB leg curl	2 × 15	(5b) RFE DB SA split squat	1 × 5 each 3 × 6 each		
		(6a) Leg tuck	2 × 5-20	(6a) RDL	1 × 5 3 × 5		
		(6b) Facepull	2 × 15	(6b) RG band pull-apart	3 × 15		
Conditioning		**Conditioning**		**Conditioning**		**Conditioning**	
2 mile run	75%-85% MHR	**6 rounds for time:**		None		None	
		(a) Fan bike	15 calories				
		(b) Hand release push-up	× 10				

Five-Day Program, Phase 1

Table 12.20   Five-Day Program, Phase 1

WEEK 1

Day 1		Day 2		Day 3		Day 4		Day 5	
(1) Vertical jump	2 × 5 (SR)	(1a) Pull-up	2 × 5 / 3 × 10	(1) High ankle hop	2 × 10 (MR)	(1) Vertical jump	2 × 5 (SR)		
(2) Squat	2 × 5 / 3 × 10	(1b) Shoulder press	2 × 5 / 3 × 10	(2) Power skip	2 × 4 each	(2a) Deadlift	2 × 5		
(3a) DB walking lunge	1 × 8 each / 3 × 12 each	(2a) SA DB bent-over row	1 × 8 each / 3 × 12 each	(3) 40 yd build-ups	× 4	(2b) Push-up	2 × 10		
(3b) Half kneeling KB chop/lift	3 × 6 each	(2b) SA DB bench press	1 × 8 each / 3 × 12 each			(3) **EMOM circuit:**	15 min		
(4a) SB leg curl	3 × 12	(3a) Hammer curl	3 × 12			(a) Deadlift	× 2 @ 74% of ACFT MDL weight		
(4b) Ab rollout	3 × 12	(3b) Rear deltoid raise	3 × 12			(b) Push-up	15% of ACFT HRP reps		
(4c) Skull crusher	3 × 12	(3c) Front plank	3 × 30 sec			(4a) Inverted row	3 × 12		
						(4b) Reverse crunch	3 × 12		
						(5a) Facepull	3 × 12		
						(5b) Side bend	3 × 12 each		
Conditioning		**Conditioning**		**Conditioning**		**Conditioning**		**Conditioning**	
100 yd shuttle (in 25 yd increments)	× 6 with 2:30 rest	None		3-5 mile run	70%-80% MHR	None		5-6 mile ruck	70%-80% MHR

Five-Day Program, Phase 1

WEEK 2

Day 1		Day 2		Day 3		Day 4	
(1) Vertical jump	2 × 5 (SR) 1 × 5 (MR)	(1a) Pull-up	2 × 5 3 × 10	(1) High ankle hop	2 × 10 (MR)	(1) Vertical jump	2 × 5 (SR)
(2) Squat	2 × 5 3 × 10	(1b) Shoulder press	2 × 5 3 × 10	(2) Power skip	2 × 4 each	(2a) Deadlift	2 × 5
(3a) DB walking lunge	1 × 8 each 3 × 12 each	(2a) SA DB bent-over row	1 × 8 each 3 × 12 each	(3) 40 yd build-ups	× 4	(2b) Push-up	2 × 10
(3b) Half kneeling KB chop/lift	3 × 6 each	(2b) SA DB bench press	1 × 8 each 3 × 12 each			(3) **EMOM circuit:**	20 min
(4a) SB leg curl	3 × 12	(3a) Hammer curl	3 × 12			(a) Deadlift	× 2 @ 74% of ACFT MDL weight
(4b) Ab rollout	3 × 12	(3b) Rear deltoid raise	3 × 12			(b) Push-up	15% of ACFT HRP reps
(4c) Skull crusher	3 × 12	(3c) Front plank	3 × 35 sec			(4a) Inverted row	3 × 12
						(4b) Reverse crunch	3 × 12
						(5a) Facepull	3 × 12
						(5b) Side bend	3 × 12 each
Conditioning		**Conditioning**		**Conditioning**		**Conditioning**	
100 yd shuttle (in 25 yd increments)	× 6 with 2:30 rest	None		3-5 mile run	70%-80% MHR	None	

Day 5	
Conditioning	
5-6 mile ruck	70%-80% MHR

(continued)

Five-Day Program, Phase 1

Table 12.20   Five-Day Program, Phase 1 (continued)

WEEK 3				
Day 1	**Day 2**	**Day 3**	**Day 4**	**Day 5**
(1) Vertical jump — 1 × 5 (SR), 2 × 5 (MR)	(1a) Pull-up — 2 × 5, 4 × 10	(1) High ankle hop — 2 × 10 (MR)	(1) Vertical jump — 2 × 5 (SR)	
(2) Squat — 2 × 5, 4 × 10	(1b) Shoulder press — 2 × 5, 4 × 10	(2) Power skip — 2 × 4 each	(2a) Deadlift — 2 × 5	
(3a) DB walking lunge — 1 × 8 each, 4 × 12 each	(2a) SA DB bent-over row — 1 × 8 each, 4 × 12 each	(3) 40 yd build-ups — × 4	(2b) Push-up — 2 × 10	
(3b) Half kneeling KB chop/lift — 3 × 6 each	(2b) SA DB bench press — 1 × 8 each, 4 × 12 each		(3) **EMOM circuit:** — 25 min	
(4a) SB leg curl — 3 × 12	(3a) Hammer curl — 4 × 12		(a) Deadlift — × 2 @ 74% of ACFT MDL weight	
(4b) Ab rollout — 3 × 12	(3b) Rear deltoid raise — 4 × 12		(b) Push-up — 15% of ACFT HRP reps	
(4c) Skull crusher — 3 × 12	(3c) Front plank — 4 × 40 sec		(4a) Inverted row — 4 × 12	
			(4b) Reverse crunch — 4 × 15	
			(5a) Facepull — 4 × 12	
			(5b) Side bend — 4 × 12 each	
Conditioning	**Conditioning**	**Conditioning**	**Conditioning**	**Conditioning**
100 yd shuttle (in 25 yd increments) — × 6 with 2:30 rest	None	3-5 mile run — 70%-80% MHR	None	5-6 mile ruck — 70%-80% MHR

Five-Day Program, Phase 1

WEEK 4

Day 1		Day 2		Day 3		Day 4		Day 5	
(1) Vertical jump	2 × 5 (SR)	(1a) Pull-up	2 × 5 / 3 × 10	(1) High ankle hop	2 × 10 (MR)	(1) Vertical jump	2 × 5 (SR)		
(2) Squat	2 × 5 / 3 × 10	(1b) Shoulder press	2 × 5 / 3 × 10	(2) Power skip	2 × 4 each	(2a) Deadlift	2 × 5		
(3a) DB walking lunge	1 × 8 each / 3 × 12 each	(2a) SA DB bent-over row	1 × 8 each / 3 × 12 each	(3) 40 yd build-ups	× 4	(2b) Push-up	2 × 10		
(3b) Half kneeling KB chop/lift	3 × 12	(2b) SA DB bench press	1 × 8 each / 3 × 12 each			(3) **EMOM circuit:**	25 min		
(4a) SB leg curl	3 × 12	(3a) Hammer curl	3 × 12			(a) Deadlift	× 2 @ 74% of ACFT MDL weight		
(4b) Ab rollout	3 × 12	(3b) Rear deltoid raise	3 × 12			(b) Push-up	15% of ACFT HRP reps		
(4c) Skull crusher	3 × 12	(3c) Front plank	3 × 30 sec			(4a) Inverted row	3 × 12		
						(4b) Reverse crunch	3 × 12		
						(5a) Facepull	3 × 12		
						(5b) Side bend	3 × 12 each		
Conditioning		**Conditioning**		**Conditioning**		**Conditioning**		**Conditioning**	
100 yd shuttle (in 25 yd increments)	× 6 with 2:30 rest	None		3-5 mile run	70%-80% MHR	None		5-6 mile ruck	70%-80% MHR

Five-Day Program, Phase 2

Table 12.21　Five-Day Program, Phase 2

WEEK 1				
Day 1	**Day 2**	**Day 3**	**Day 4**	**Day 5**
(1) Vertical jump — 1 × 5 (SR), 2 × 5 (MR)	(1a) Chin-up — 2 × 5, 4 × 8	(1) High ankle hop — 2 × 10 (MR)	(1a) Deadbug arm only — 2 × 5 each	
(2) MB scoop toss — 3 × 5	(1b) Shoulder press — 2 × 5, 4 × 8	(2) Power skip — 2 × 4 each	(1b) Deadbug leg only — 2 × 5 each	
(3) Deadlift — 2 × 5, 4 × 5	(2a) DB bent-over row — 1 × 5, 3 × 15	(3) 40 yd build-ups — × 6	(2) Vertical jump — 2 × 5 (SR), 1 × 5 (MR)	
(4a) DB lunge — 1 × 10 each, 3 × 15 each	(2b) SA DB incline bench — 1 × 5 each, 3 × 15 each		(3a) RDL — 2 × 5, 4 × 5 (ECC3)	
(4b) Lying trunk twist — 3 × 8 each	(3a) DB biceps curl — 3 × 15		(3b) Facepull — 4 × 15	
(5a) SB leg curl — 3 × 15	(3b) Band pull-apart — 3 × 15		(4) **EMOM circuit:** — 20 min	
(5b) Ab rollout — 3 × 15	(3c) Wtd plank — 3 × 30 sec		(a) Pull-up — × 2	
(5c) Triceps pushdown — 3 × 12-15			(b) Push-up — × 4	
			(c) Sit-up — × 4	
			(d) Squat — × 4	
Conditioning	**Conditioning**	**Conditioning**	**Conditioning**	**Conditioning**
150 yd shuttle (in 25 yd increments) — × 6 with 2:30 rest	None	3-5 mile run — 75%-85% MHR	Fan bike — 4 × 30 sec with 4 min rest	5-6 mile ruck — 75%-85% MHR

Five-Day Program, Phase 2

WEEK 2

Day 1		Day 2		Day 3		Day 4		Day 5	
(1) Vertical jump	1 × 5 (SR) 2 × 5 (MR)	(1a) Chin-up	2 × 5 4 × 8	(1) High ankle hop	2 × 10 (MR)	(1a) Deadbug arm only	2 × 6 each		
(2) MB scoop toss	3 × 5	(1b) Shoulder press	2 × 5 4 × 8	(2) Power skip	2 × 4 each	(1b) Deadbug leg only	2 × 6 each		
(3) Deadlift	2 × 5 5 × 5	(2a) DB bent-over row	1 × 5 3 × 15	(3) 40 yd build-ups	× 6	(2) Vertical jump	1 × 5 (SR) 2 × 5 (MR)		
(4a) DB lunge	1 × 10 each 3 × 15 each	(2b) SA DB incline bench	1 × 5 each 3 × 15 each			(3a) RDL	2 × 5 4 × 5 (ECC3)		
(4b) Lying trunk twist	3 × 8 each	(3a) DB biceps curl	3 × 15			(3b) Facepull	4 × 15		
(5a) SB leg curl	3 × 15	(3b) Band pull-apart	3 × 15			(4) **EMOM circuit:**	20 min		
(5b) Ab rollout	3 × 15	(3c) Wtd plank	3 × 30 sec			(a) Pull-up	× 2		
(5c) Triceps pushdown	3 × 12-15					(b) Push-up	× 4		
						(c) Sit-up	× 4		
						(d) Squat	× 4		
Conditioning		**Conditioning**		**Conditioning**		**Conditioning**		**Conditioning**	
150 yd shuttle (in 25 yd increments)	× 6 with 2:30 rest	None		3-5 mile run	75%-85% MHR	Fan bike	4 × 30 sec with 4 min rest	5-6 mile ruck	75%-85% MHR

(continued)

Five-Day Program, Phase 2

Table 12.21   Five-Day Program, Phase 2 (continued)

WEEK 3

Day 1		Day 2		Day 3		Day 4		Day 5	
(1) Vertical jump	1 × 5 (SR) 2 × 5 (MR)	(1a) Chin-up	2 × 5 4 × 8	(1) High ankle hop	2 × 10 (MR)	(1a) Deadbug arm only	2 × 8 each		
(2) MB scoop toss	3 × 5	(1b) Shoulder press	2 × 5 4 × 8	(2) Power skip	2 × 4 each	(1b) Deadbug leg only	2 × 8 each		
(3) Deadlift	2 × 5 5 × 5	(2a) DB bent-over row	1 × 5 3 × 15	(3) 40 yd build-ups	× 6	(2) Vertical jump	1 × 5 (SR) 2 × 5 (MR)		
(4a) DB lunge	1 × 10 each 3 × 15 each	(2b) SA DB incline bench	1 × 5 each 3 × 15 each			(3a) RDL	2 × 5 4 × 5 (ECC3)		
(4b) Lying trunk twist	4 × 8 each	(3a) DB biceps curl	3 × 15			(3b) Facepull	4 × 15		
(5a) SB leg curl	3 × 15	(3b) Band pull-apart	3 × 15			(4) **EMOM circuit:**	20 min		
(5b) Ab rollout	3 × 15	(3c) Wtd plank	3 × 30 sec			(a) Pull-up	× 3		
(5c) Triceps pushdown	3 × 12-15					(b) Push-up	× 5		
						(c) Sit-up	× 5		
						(d) Squat	× 7		
Conditioning		**Conditioning**		**Conditioning**		**Conditioning**		**Conditioning**	
150 yd shuttle (in 25 yd increments)	× 6 with 2:30 rest	None		3-5 mile run	75%-85% MHR	Fan bike	4 × 30 sec with 3 min rest	5-6 mile ruck	75%-85% MHR

WEEK 4

Day 1		Day 2		Day 3		Day 4		Day 5	
(1) Vertical jump	1 × 5 (SR) 2 × 5 (MR)	(1a) Chin-up	2 × 5 3 × 8	(1) High ankle hop	2 × 10 (MR)	(1a) Deadbug arm only	2 × 8 each		
(2) MB scoop toss	3 × 5	(1b) Shoulder press	2 × 5 3 × 8	(2) Power skip	2 × 4 each	(1b) Deadbug leg only	2 × 8 each		
(3) Deadlift	2 × 5 4 × 5	(2a) DB bent-over row	1 × 5 3 × 15	(3) 40 yd build-ups	× 6	(2) Vertical jump	1 × 5 (SR) 2 × 5 (MR)		
(4a) DB lunge	1 × 10 each 3 × 15 each	(2b) SA DB incline bench	1 × 5 each 3 × 15 each			(3a) RDL	2 × 5 3 × 8		
(4b) Lying trunk twist	4 × 8 each	(3a) DB biceps curl	3 × 15			(3b) Facepull	4 × 15		
(5a) SB leg curl	3 × 15	(3b) Band pull-apart	3 × 15			(4) **EMOM circuit:**	20 min		
(5b) Ab rollout	3 × 15	(3c) Wtd plank	3 × 30 sec			(a) Pull-up	× 3		
(5c) Triceps pushdown	3 × 12-15					(b) Push-up	× 5		
						(c) Sit-up	× 5		
						(d) Squat	× 7		
Conditioning		**Conditioning**		**Conditioning**		**Conditioning**		**Conditioning**	
150 yd shuttle (in 25 yd increments)	× 6 with 2:30 rest	None		3-5 mile run	75%-85% MHR	Fan bike	4 × 30 sec with 3 min rest	5-6 mile ruck	75%-85% MHR

Table 12.22   Five-Day Program, Phase 3

WEEK 1

Day 1		Day 2		Day 3		Day 4		Day 5	
(1) Lateral bound	3 × 4 each (SR)	(1) High ankle hop	2 × 10 (MR)	(1) Vertical jump	3 × 5 (SR)	(1) High ankle hop	2 × 10 (MR)	(1) Deadbug	2 × 8 each
(2) Squat	2 × 5 4 × 5	(2) Power skip	2 × 4 each	(2) MB scoop toss	3 × 5	(2) Power skip	2 × 4 each	(2a) Broad jump	3 × 3 (SR)
(3a) Bent-over row	1 × 5 4 × 5	(3) 40 yd build-ups	× 6	(3) Deadlift	2 × 5 4 × 5	(3) 40 yd build-ups	× 6	(2b) Chin-up	1 × 5 4 × 5
(3b) DB incline press	1 × 5 4 × 10			(4a) Alt DB prone row	1 × 5 each 4 × 10 each			(3a) Shoulder press	2 × 5 4 × 5
(4a) SA/SL DB RDL	3 × 10 each			(4b) Glute-ham raise	4 × 10			(3b) DB reverse lunge	1 × 5 each 4 × 10 each
(4b) Rear deltoid raise	3 × 10			(4c) Sit-up	4 × 20			(4a) RDL	1 × 5 4 × 5 (ISO3)
(4c) Ab rollout	3 × 10			(5a) Bench press	2 × 5 4 × 5			(4b) Band pull-apart	4 × 15
				(5b) Facepull	4 × 15			(4c) Stir the pot	4 × 3 each with 4 sec circles
				(5c) Pallof press	4 × 5 each side (ECC5)				
Conditioning		**Conditioning**		**Conditioning**		**Conditioning**		**Conditioning**	
Rower time trial	500 m × 3 with 5 min rest	1 mile repeats	× 3 at 2-mile pace with 1:1 W:R ratio	15 min timed block:	AMRAP	3-5 mile run	75%-85% MHR	Fan bike	4 × 30 sec with 3 min rest
				(a) 30 yd Sled push (in 15 yd increments)					
				(b) 30 yd DB farmer walk (in 15 yd increments)					

WEEK 2

Day 1

Exercise	Sets × Reps
(1) Lateral bound	3 × 4 each (SR)
(2) Squat	2 × 5, 4 × 5
(3a) Bent-over row	1 × 5, 4 × 5
(3b) DB incline press	1 × 5, 4 × 10
(4a) SA/SL DB RDL	3 × 10 each
(4b) Rear deltoid raise	3 × 10
(4c) Ab rollout	3 × 10
Conditioning	
Rower time trial	500 m × 3 with 5 min rest

Day 2

Exercise	Sets × Reps
(1) High ankle hop	2 × 10 (MR)
(2) Power skip	2 × 4 each
(3) 40 yd build-ups	× 6
Conditioning	
1 mile repeats	× 3 at 2-mile pace with 1:1 W:R ratio

Day 3

Exercise	Sets × Reps
(1) Vertical jump	3 × 5 (SR)
(2) MB scoop toss	3 × 5
(3) Deadlift	2 × 5, 4 × 5
(4a) Alt DB prone row	1 × 5 each, 4 × 10 each
(4b) Glute-ham raise	4 × 10
(4c) Sit-up	4 × 20
(5a) Bench press	2 × 5, 4 × 5
(5b) Facepull	4 × 15
(5c) Pallof press	4 × 5 each side (ECC5)
Conditioning	
15 min timed block:	AMRAP
(a) 30 yd Sled push (in 15 yd increments)	
(b) 30 yd DB farmer walk (in 15 yd increments)	

Day 4

Exercise	Sets × Reps
(1) High ankle hop	2 × 10 (MR)
(2) Power skip	2 × 4 each
(3) 40 yd build-ups	× 6
Conditioning	
5-6 mile ruck	75%-85% MHR

Day 5

Exercise	Sets × Reps
(1) Deadbug	2 × 8 each
(2a) Broad jump	3 × 3 (SR)
(2b) Chin-up	1 × 5, 4 × 5
(3a) Shoulder press	2 × 5, 4 × 5
(3b) DB reverse lunge	1 × 5 each, 4 × 10 each
(4a) RDL	1 × 5, 4 × 5 (ISO3)
(4b) Band pull-apart	4 × 15
(4c) Stir the pot	4 × 5 each with 4 sec circles
Conditioning	
Fan bike	5 × 30 sec with 3 min rest

(continued)

Table 12.22 Five-Day Program, Phase 3 (continued)

WEEK 3

Day 1

Exercise	Sets × reps
(1) Lateral bound	3 × 4 each (SR)
(2) Squat	2 × 5 4 × 4
(3a) Bent-over row	1 × 5 4 × 4
(3b) DB incline press	1 × 5 4 × 8
(4a) SA/SL DB RDL	3 × 8 each
(4b) Rear deltoid raise	3 × 10
(4c) Ab rollout	3 × 10
Conditioning	
Rower time trial	500 m × 3 with 5 min rest

Day 2

Exercise	Sets × reps
(1) High ankle hop	2 × 10 (MR)
(2) Power skip	2 × 4 each
(3) 40 yd build-ups	× 6
Conditioning	
1 mile repeats	× 3 at 2-mile pace with 1:1 W:R ratio

Day 3

Exercise	Sets × reps
(1) Vertical jump	3 × 5 (SR)
(2) MB scoop toss	3 × 5
(3) Deadlift	2 × 5 4 × 3
(4a) Alt DB prone row	1 × 5 each 4 × 8 each
(4b) Glute-ham raise	4 × 10
(4c) Sit-up	4 × 25
(5a) Bench press	2 × 5 4 × 3
(5b) Facepull	4 × 15
(5c) Pallof press	4 × 10 each side (ECC3)
Conditioning	
15 min timed block:	AMRAP
(a) 30 yd Sled push (in 15 yd increments)	
(b) 30 yd DB farmer walk (in 15 yd increments)	

Day 4

Exercise	Sets × reps
(1) High ankle hop	2 × 10 (MR)
(2) Power skip	2 × 4 each
(3) 40 yd build-ups	× 6
Conditioning	
3-5 mile run	75%-85% MHR

Day 5

Exercise	Sets × reps
(1) Deadbug	3 × 8 each
(2a) Broad jump	3 × 3 (SR)
(2b) Chin-up	1 × 5 4 × 3
(3a) Shoulder press	2 × 5 4 × 3
(3b) DB reverse lunge	1 × 5 each 4 × 8 each
(4a) RDL	1 × 5 4 × 5 (ISO3)
(4b) Band pull-apart	4 × 15
(4c) Stir the pot	4 × 5 each with 4 sec circles
Conditioning	
Fan bike	5 × 30 sec with 3 min rest

Five-Day Program, Phase 3

WEEK 4

Day 1

Exercise	Sets × Reps
(1) Lateral bound	3 × 4 each (SR)
(2) Squat	2 × 5 / 4 × 3
(3a) Bent-over row	1 × 5 / 3 × 4
(3b) DB incline press	1 × 5 / 4 × 8
(4a) SA/SL DB RDL	3 × 8 each
(4b) Rear deltoid raise	3 × 10
(4c) Ab rollout	3 × 10

Conditioning

Rower time trial	500 m × 3 with 5 min rest

Day 2

Exercise	Sets × Reps
(1) High ankle hop	2 × 10 (MR)
(2) Power skip	2 × 4 each
(3) 40 yd build-ups	× 6

Conditioning

1 mile repeats	× 3 at 2-mile pace with 1:1 W:R ratio

Day 3

Exercise	Sets × Reps
(1) Vertical jump	3 × 5 (SR)
(2) MB scoop toss	2 × 5
(3) Deadlift	2 × 5 / 4 × 3
(4a) Alt DB prone row	1 × 5 each / 3 × 8 each
(4b) Glute-ham raise	3 × 10
(4c) Sit-up	3 × 25
(5a) Bench press	2 × 5 / 3 × 3
(5b) Facepull	3 × 15
(5c) Pallof press	4 × 10 each side (ECC3)

Conditioning

15 min timed block:	AMRAP
(a) 30 yd Sled push (in 15 yd increments)	
(b) 30 yd DB farmer walk (in 15 yd increments)	

Day 4

Exercise	Sets × Reps
(1) High ankle hop	2 × 10 (MR)
(2) Power skip	2 × 4 each
(3) 40 yd build-ups	× 6

Conditioning

5-6 mile ruck	75%-85% MHR

Day 5

Exercise	Sets × Reps
(1) Deadbug	3 × 8 each
(2a) Broad jump	3 × 3 (SR)
(2b) Chin-up	1 × 5 / 4 × 3
(3a) Shoulder press	2 × 5 / 4 × 3
(3b) DB reverse lunge	1 × 5 each / 3 × 8 each
(4a) RDL	1 × 5 / 3 × 5
(4b) Band pull-apart	3 × 15
(4c) Stir the pot	4 × 5 each with 4 sec circles

Conditioning

Fan bike	5 × 30 sec with 3 min rest

Five-Day Program, Phase 4

Table 12.23 Five-Day Program, Phase 4

	WEEK 1				
	Day 1	**Day 2**	**Day 3**	**Day 4**	**Day 5**
	(1) Lateral bound — 1 × 4 each (SR), 2 × 4 each (MR)	(1) High ankle hop — 2 × 10 (MR)	(1) Vertical jump — 1 × 5 (SR), 2 × 5 (MR)	(1) High ankle hop — 2 × 10 (MR)	(1) Broad jump — 1 × 3 (SR), 2 × 3 (MR)
	(2) DB quarter squat jump — 1 × 5 (SR), 2 × 5 (SR)	(2) Bound — 2 × 4 each (SR)	(2) Tuck jump — 2 × 5 (MR)	(2) Power skip — 2 × 4 each	(2) Hang clean low pull — 1 × 5, 2 × 5
	(3) Squat — 2 × 5, 4 × 5	(3) Power skip — 2 × 4 each	(3a) Deadlift — 2 × 5, 4 × 5	(3) 40 yd build-ups — × 6	(3) Pull-up — 1 × 5, 4 × 5
	(4a) RG bent-over row — 1 × 5, 4 × 5	(4) 40 yd build-ups — × 6	(3b) MB scoop toss — 4 × 5		(4a) Shoulder press — 2 × 5, 4 × 5
	(4b) Wtd push-up — 1 × 10, 4 × 10		(4a) DB prone row — 1 × 5, 4 × 10		(4b) DB lunge — 1 × 5 each, 4 × 10 each
	(5a) DB SL RDL — 3 × 10 each		(4b) Poor man's glute-ham raise — 4 × 5		(5a) RDL — 1 × 5, 4 × 5
	(5b) Facepull — 3 × 15		(5a) Bench press — 2 × 5, 4 × 5		(5b) Rear deltoid raise — 3 × 10
	(5c) Hanging knee raise — 3 × 12		(5b) RG band pullapart — 4 × 15		(5c) Eccentric dragon flag — 3 × 10
			(5c) Ab rollout — 3 × 12		
Conditioning	Conditioning	Conditioning	Conditioning	Conditioning	Conditioning
	150 yd shuttle (in 25 yd increments) — × 5 with 1:30 rest	400 m repeats — × 9 at 5%-15% faster than 2-mile pace with 1:1 W:R ratio	Rower time trial — 500 m × 3 with 1:3 W:R ratio	3-5 mile run — 75%-85% MHR	**8 rounds for time:**
					(a) Fan bike — 15 calories
					(b) Hand release push-up — × 10

Five-Day Program, Phase 4

WEEK 2

Day 1

Exercise	Prescription
(1) Lateral bound	1 × 4 each (SR) / 2 × 4 each (MR)
(2) DB quarter squat jump	1 × 5 (SR) / 2 × 5 (SR)
(3) Squat	2 × 5 / 4 × 3
(4a) RG bent-over row	1 × 5 / 4 × 5
(4b) Wtd push-up	1 × 10 / 4 × 8
(5a) DB SL RDL	3 × 8 each
(5b) Facepull	3 × 15
(5c) Hanging knee raise	3 × 15

Conditioning

Exercise	Prescription
150 yd shuttle (in 25 yd increments)	× 5 with 1:30 rest

Day 2

Exercise	Prescription
(1) High ankle hop	2 × 10 (MR)
(2) Bound	2 × 4 each (SR)
(3) Power skip	2 × 4 each
(4) 40 yd build-ups	× 6

Conditioning

Exercise	Prescription
400 m repeats	× 9 at 5%-15% faster than 2-mile pace with 1:1 W:R ratio

Day 3

Exercise	Prescription
(1) Vertical jump	1 × 5 (SR) / 2 × 5 (MR)
(2) Tuck jump	2 × 5 (MR)
(3a) Deadlift	2 × 5 / 4 × 3
(3b) MB scoop toss	3 × 5
(4a) DB prone row	1 × 5 / 4 × 8
(4b) Poor man's glute-ham raise	4 × 5
(5a) Bench press	2 × 5 / 4 × 3
(5b) RG band pullapart	4 × 15
(5c) Ab rollout	3 × 12

Conditioning

Exercise	Prescription
Rower time trial	500 m × 3 with 1:3 W:R ratio

Day 4

Exercise	Prescription
(1) High ankle hop	2 × 10 (MR)
(2) Power skip	2 × 4 each
(3) 40 yd build-ups	× 6

Conditioning

Exercise	Prescription
5-6 mile ruck	75%-85% MHR

Day 5

Exercise	Prescription
(1) Broad jump	1 × 3 (SR) / 2 × 3 (MR)
(2) Hang clean low pull	1 × 5 / 3 × 5
(3) Pull-up	1 × 5 / 4 × 3
(4a) Shoulder press	2 × 5 / 4 × 3
(4b) DB lunge	1 × 5 each / 4 × 8 each
(5a) RDL	1 × 5 / 4 × 5
(5b) Rear deltoid raise	3 × 10
(5c) Eccentric dragon flag	3 × 10

Conditioning

8 rounds for time:

Exercise	Prescription
(a) Fan bike	15 calories
(b) Hand release push-up	× 10

(continued)

Five-Day Program, Phase 4

Table 12.23 Five-Day Program, Phase 4 (continued)

WEEK 3

	Day 1	Day 2	Day 3	Day 4	Day 5
(1)	Lateral bound: 1 × 4 each (SR), 2 × 4 each (MR)	(1) High ankle hop: 2 × 10 (MR)	(1) Vertical jump: 1 × 5 (SR), 2 × 5 (MR)	(1) High ankle hop: 2 × 10 (MR)	(1) Broad jump: 1 × 3 (SR), 2 × 3 (MR)
(2)	DB quarter squat jump: 1 × 5 (SR), 2 × 5 (SR)	(2) Bound: 2 × 4 each (SR)	(2) Tuck jump: 2 × 5 (MR)	(2) Power skip: 2 × 4 each	(2) Hang clean low pull: 1 × 5, 3 × 5
(3)	Squat: 2 × 5, 4 × 3,2,1,1	(3) Power skip: 2 × 4 each	(3a) Deadlift: 2 × 5, 4 × 3	(3) 40 yd build-ups: × 6	(3) Pull-up: 1 × 5, 4 × 3,2,2,2
	(4a) RG bent-over row: 1 × 5, 4 × 4	(4) 40 yd build-ups: × 6	(3b) MB scoop toss: 3 × 5		(4a) Shoulder press: 2 × 5, 4 × 3,2,2,2
	(4b) Wtd push-up: 1 × 10, 4 × 8		(4a) DB prone row: 1 × 5, 4 × 8		(4b) DB lunge: 1 × 5 each, 4 × 8 each
	(5a) DB SL RDL: 3 × 8 each		(4b) Poor man's glute-ham raise: 4 × 6		(5a) RDL: 1 × 5, 4 × 5
	(5b) Facepull: 3 × 15		(5a) Bench press: 2 × 5, 4 × 3,2,1,1		(5b) Rear deltoid raise: 3 × 10
	(5c) Hanging knee raise: 3 × 15		(5b) RG band pullapart: 4 × 15		(5c) Eccentric dragon flag: 3 × 10
			(5c) Ab rollout: 3 × 15		
Conditioning	150 yd shuttle (in 25 yd increments): × 5 with 1:30 rest	400 m repeats: × 9 at 5%-15% faster than 2-mile pace with 1:1 W:R ratio	Rower time trial: 500 m × 3 with 1:3 W:R ratio	3-5 mile run: 75%-85% MHR	8 rounds for time: (a) Fan bike: 15 calories; (b) Hand release push-up: × 10

WEEK 4

Day 1		Day 2		Day 3		Day 4		Day 5	
(1) Lateral bound	1 × 4 each (SR) / 2 × 4 each (MR)	(1) High ankle hop	2 × 10 (MR)	(1) Vertical jump	1 × 5 (SR) / 2 × 5 (MR)	(1) High ankle hop	2 × 10 (MR)	(1) Broad jump	1 × 3 (SR) / 2 × 3 (MR)
(2) DB quarter squat jump	1 × 5 (SR) / 2 × 5 (SR)	(2) Bound	2 × 4 each (SR)	(2) Tuck jump	2 × 5 (MR)	(2) Power skip	2 × 4 each	(2) Hang clean low pull	1 × 5 / 3 × 5
(3) Squat	2 × 5 / 3 × 3	(3) Power skip	2 × 4 each	(3a) Deadlift	2 × 5 / 4 × 3,2,1,1	(3) 40 yd build-ups	× 6	(3) Pull-up	1 × 5 / 3 × 3
(4a) RG bent-over row	1 × 5 / 3 × 4	(4) 40 yd build-ups	× 6	(3b) MB scoop toss	2 × 4			(4a) Shoulder press	2 × 5 / 3 × 3
(4b) Wtd push-up	1 × 10 / 3 × 8			(4a) DB prone row	1 × 5 / 3 × 8			(4b) DB lunge	1 × 5 each / 3 × 8 each
(5a) DB SL RDL	3 × 8 each			(4b) Poor man's glute-ham raise	3 × 5			(5a) RDL	1 × 5 / 3 × 5
(5b) Facepull	3 × 15			(5a) Bench press	2 × 5 / 3 × 3			(5b) Rear deltoid raise	3 × 10
(5c) Hanging knee raise	3 × 15			(5b) RG band pullapart	4 × 15			(5c) Eccentric dragon flag	3 × 10
				(5c) Ab rollout	3 × 15				
Conditioning		**Conditioning**		**Conditioning**		**Conditioning**		**Conditioning**	
150 yd shuttle (in 25 yd increments)	× 5 with 1:30 rest	400 m repeats	× 9 at 5%-15% faster than 2-mile pace with 1:1 W:R ratio	Rower time trial	500 m × 3 with 1:3 W:R ratio	5-6 mile ruck	75%-85% MHR	**8 rounds for time:**	
								(a) Fan bike	15 calories
								(b) Hand release push-up	× 10

Five-Day Program, Phase 5

Table 12.24 Five-Day Program, Phase 5

WEEK 1

Day 1

(1) Lateral bound	1 × 4 each (SR)	2 × 4 each (MR)
(2) MB scoop toss	3 × 5	
(3) Deadlift	2 × 5	6 × 5,3,1,5,3,1
(4a) DB prone row	1 × 5	4 × 10
(4b) Glute-ham raise	4 × 10	
(5a) Bench press	2 × 5	Work up to a 5RM then do 2 × 8 @ 80% of 5RM
(5b) RG band pullapart	4 × 15	
(5c) Leg tuck	4 × 5-10	
Conditioning		
Backward sled drag (25 yds) + shuttle (25 yds)	× 6 with 1:3 W:R ratio	

Day 2

(1) High ankle hop	2 × 10 (MR)
(2) Power skip	2 × 4 each
(3) Bound	1 × 4 each (SR), 2 × 4 each (MR)
(4) 40 yd build-ups	× 6
Conditioning	
800 m repeats	× 5 at 5%-15% faster than 2-mile pace with 1:1 W:R ratio

Day 3

(1) Vertical jump	1 × 5 (SR)	2 × 5 (MR)
(2) DB quarter squat jump	1 × 5 (MR)	1 × 5 (MR)
(3) Squat	2 × 5	4 × 5
(4a) RG bent-over row	1 × 5	4 × 5
(4b) Push-up on DBs	1 × 10% of ACFT HRP reps	4 × 50% of ACFT HRP reps
(5a) SL RDL	3 × 8 each	
(5b) Facepull	3 × 15	
(5c) Roman side crunch	3 × 10 each	
Conditioning		
6 rounds for time:		
(a) Rower	500 m	
(b) Hand release push-up	× 10	

Day 4

(1) High ankle hop	2 × 10 (MR)
(2) Power skip	2 × 4 each
(3) Bound	1 × 4 each (SR), 2 × 4 each (MR)
(4) 40 yd build-ups	× 6
Conditioning	
3-5 mile run	75%-85% MHR

Day 5

(1) Broad jump	1 × 3 (SR)	2 × 3 (MR)
(2) Hang clean low pull	2 × 5	3 × 5
(3) Pull-up (working sets: Wtd pull-up)	1 × 5	Work up to a 5RM then do 2 × 8 @ 80% of 5RM
(4a) Shoulder press	2 × 5	Work up to a 5RM then do 2 × 8 @ 80% of 5RM
(4b) Lateral squat	1 × 5 each	3 × 10 each
(5a) RDL	1 × 5	3 × 10
(5b) Rear deltoid raise	3 × 10	
(5c) Landmine twist	3 × 6 each	
Conditioning		
15 min timed block:	AMRAP	
(a) 30 yd Sled push (in 15 yd increments)		
(b) 30 yd DB farmer walk (in 15 yd increments)		

Five-Day Program, Phase 5

WEEK 2

	Day 1	Day 2	Day 3	Day 4	Day 5
(1)	Lateral bound — 1 × 4 each (SR); 2 × 4 each (MR)	High ankle hop — 2 × 10 (MR)	Vertical jump — 1 × 5 (SR); 2 × 5 (MR)	High ankle hop — 2 × 10 (MR)	Broad jump — 1 × 3 (SR); 2 × 3 (MR)
(2)	MB scoop toss — 3 × 5	Power skip — 2 × 4 each	DB quarter squat jump — 1 × 5 (MR); 1 × 5 (MR)	Power skip — 2 × 4 each	Hang clean low pull — 2 × 5; 3 × 5
(3)	Deadlift — 2 × 5; 6 × 5,3,1,5,3,1	Bound — 1 × 4 each (SR); 2 × 4 each (MR)	Squat — 2 × 5; 4 × 5	Bound — 1 × 4 each (SR); 2 × 4 each (MR)	Pull-up (working sets: Wtd pull-up) — 1 × 5; Work up to a 3RM then do 2 × 6 @ 80% of 3RM
(4) / (4a)	(4a) DB prone row — 1 × 5; 4 × 10	(4) 40 yd build-ups — × 6	(4a) RG bent-over row — 1 × 5; 4 × 5	(4) 40 yd build-ups — × 6	(4a) Shoulder press — 2 × 5; Work up to a 3RM then do 2 × 6 @ 80% of 3RM
(4b)	Glute-ham raise — 4 × 10		Push-up on DBs — 1 × 10% of *ACFT HRP reps*; 4 × 50% of ACFT HRP reps		Lateral squat — 1 × 5 *each*; 3 × 10 each
(5a)	Bench press — 2 × 5; Work up to a 3RM then do 2 × 6 @ 80% of 3RM		SL RDL — 3 × 8 each		RDL — 1 × 5; 3 × 10
(5b)	RG band pullapart — 4 × 15		Facepull — 3 × 15		Rear deltoid raise — 4 × 10
(5c)	Leg tuck — 4 × 5-10		Roman side crunch — 3 × 10 each		Landmine twist — 3 × 8 each
Conditioning	Backward sled drag (25 yds) + shuttle (25 yds) — × 6 with 1:3 W:R ratio	800 m repeats — × 5 at 5%-15% faster than 2-mile pace with 1:1 W:R ratio	6 rounds for time: (a) Rower — 500 m; (b) Hand release push-up — × 10	5-6 mile ruck — 75%-85% MHR	15 min timed block: — AMRAP; (a) 30 yd Sled push (in 15 yd increments); (b) 30 yd DB farmer walk (in 15 yd increments)

(continued)

Five-Day Program, Phase 5

Table 12.24 Five-Day Program, Phase 5 (continued)

WEEK 3

	Day 1	Day 2	Day 3	Day 4	Day 5
(1)	Lateral bound — 1 × 4 each (SR); 2 × 4 each (MR)	High ankle hop — 2 × 10 (MR)	Vertical jump — 1 × 5 (SR); 2 × 5 (MR)	High ankle hop — 2 × 10 (MR)	Broad jump — 1 × 3 (SR); 2 × 3 (MR)
(2)	MB scoop toss — 3 × 5	Power skip — 2 × 4 each	DB quarter squat jump — 1 × 5 (MR); 1 × 5 (MR)	Power skip — 2 × 4 each	Hang clean low pull — 2 × 5; 3 × 5
(3)	Deadlift — 2 × 5, Work up to a 3RM	Bound — 1 × 4 each (SR); 2 × 4 each (MR)	Squat — 2 × 5; 4 × 5	Bound — 1 × 4 each (SR); 2 × 4 each (MR)	Pull-up (working sets: Wtd pull-up) — 1 × 5, Work up to a 3RM then do 2 × 6 @ 80% of 3RM
(4a)/(4)	(4a) DB prone row — 1 × 5; 4 × 10	(4) 40 yd build-ups — × 6	(4a) RG bent-over row — 1 × 5; 4 × 4	(4) 40 yd build-ups — × 6	(4a) Shoulder press — 2 × 5, Work up to a 3RM then do 2 × 6 @ 80% of 3RM
(4b)	Glute-ham raise — 4 × 10		Push-up on DBs — *1 × 10% of ACFT HRP reps*; 4 × 60% of ACFT HRP reps		Lateral squat — *1 × 5 each*; 3 × 8 each
(5a)	Bench press — 2 × 5, Work up to a 1RM then do 2 × 4 @ 80% 1RM		SL RDL — 3 × 8 each		RDL — 1 × 5; 3 × 8
(5b)	RG band pullapart — 4 × 10		Facepull — 3 × 15		Rear deltoid raise — 4 × 10
(5c)	Leg tuck — 4 × 5-15		Roman side crunch — 3 × 15 each		Landmine twist — 3 × 10 each
Conditioning	Backward sled drag (25 yds) + shuttle (25 yds) — × 6 with 1:3 W:R ratio	800 m repeats — × 5 at 5%-15% faster than 2-mile pace with 1:1 W:R ratio	**6 rounds for time:** (a) Rower — 500 m; (b) Hand release push-up — × 10	3-5 mile run — 75%-85% MHR	**15 min timed block:** AMRAP (a) 30 yd Sled push (in 15 yd increments); (b) 30 yd DB farmer walk (in 15 yd increments)

WEEK 4

Day 1

Exercise	Sets × Reps
(1) Lateral bound	1 × 4 each (SR) / 2 × 4 each (MR)
(2) MB scoop toss	3 × 5
(3) Deadlift	2 × 5 / 3 × 3
(4a) DB prone row	1 × 5 / 3 × 10
(4b) Glute-ham raise	3 × 10
(5a) Bench press	2 × 5 / 3 × 5
(5b) RG band pullapart	4 × 10
(5c) Leg tuck	4 × 5-15

Conditioning

Backward sled drag (25 yds) + shuttle (25 yds): × 6 with 1:3 W:R ratio

Day 2

Exercise	Sets × Reps
(1) High ankle hop	2 × 10 (MR)
(2) Power skip	2 × 4 each
(3) Bound	1 × 4 each (SR) / 2 × 4 each (MR)
(4) 40 yd build-ups	× 6

Conditioning

1 mile time trial; Rest 10 minutes; 800 m repeats: × 2 at 5%-15% faster than 2-mile pace with 1:1 W:R ratio

Day 3

Exercise	Sets × Reps
(1) Vertical jump	1 × 5 (SR) / 2 × 5 (MR)
(2) DB quarter squat jump	1 × 5 (MR) / 1 × 5 (MR)
(3) Squat	2 × 5 / 3 × 5
(4a) RG bent-over row	1 × 5 / 4 × 4
(4b) Push-up on DBs	1 × 10% of ACFT HRP reps / 3 × 60% of ACFT HRP reps
(4a) SL RDL	3 × 8 each
(4b) Facepull	3 × 15
(4c) Roman side crunch	3 × 15 each

Conditioning

6 rounds for time:
- (a) Rower: 500 m
- (b) Hand release push-up: × 10

Day 4

Exercise	Sets × Reps
(1) High ankle hop	2 × 10 (MR)
(2) Power skip	2 × 4 each
(3) Bound	1 × 4 each (SR) / 2 × 4 each (MR)
(4) 40 yd build-ups	× 6

Conditioning

5-6 mile ruck: 75%-85% MHR

Day 5

Exercise	Sets × Reps
(1) Broad jump	1 × 3 (SR) / 2 × 3 (MR)
(2) Hang clean low pull	2 × 5 / 3 × 5
(3) Pull-up	1 × 5 / 3 × 3
(4a) Shoulder press	2 × 5 / 3 × 3
(4b) Lateral squat	1 × 5 each / 3 × 8 each
(5a) RDL	1 × 5 / 3 × 8
(5b) Rear deltoid raise	4 × 10
(5c) Landmine twist	3 × 10 each

Conditioning

15 min timed block: AMRAP
- (a) 30 yd Sled push (in 15 yd increments)
- (b) 30 yd DB farmer walk (in 15 yd increments)

Five-Day Program, Phase 6

Table 12.25   Five-Day Program, Phase 6

WEEK 1

Day 1		Day 2		Day 3		Day 4		Day 5	
(1) High ankle hop	2 × 10 (MR)	(1) Broad jump	1 × 3 (SR) 2 × 3 (MR)	(1) Vertical jump	1 × 5 (SR) 2 × 5 (MR)	(1) High ankle hop	2 × 10 (MR)	(1) High ankle hop	1 × 10 (MR)
(2) Power skip	2 × 4 each	(2) Lateral bound	1 × 4 each (SR) 2 × 4 each (MR)	(2) 50 yd shuttle with alt foot plant	× 6	(2) Power skip	2 × 4 each	(2) Vertical jump	1 × 5 (SR)
(3) Bound	1 × 4 each (SR) 2 × 4 each (MR)	(3) MB scoop toss	3 × 5	(3) Hang clean low pull	2 × 5 4 × 3			(3) Power skip	2 × 4 each
(4) 40 yd build-ups	× 6	(4a) Chin-up	2 × 5 4 × 8,6,6 1 × AMRAP (>5 reps)	(4a) Inverted row	1 × 5 4 × 10			(4) ACFT practice	90% of previous ACFT results
		(4b) Lateral squat	1 × 5 each 4 × 5 each	(4b) Body saw	4 × 10				
		(5a) Incline bench press	2 × 5 4 × 8,6,6	(5a) SA DB shoulder press	1 × 5 each 4 × 10 each				
		(5b) SB leg curl	4 × 15	(5b) RFE DB SA split squat	1 × 5 each 4 × 10 each				
		(6a) Leg tuck	4 × 5-20	(6a) RDL	1 × 5 3 × 5 1 × 10				
		(6b) Facepull	4 × 15	(6b) RG band pullapart	4 × 15				
Conditioning		**Conditioning**		**Conditioning**		**Conditioning**		**Conditioning**	
400 m repeats	× 9 at 5%-15% faster than 1-mile pace with 1:1 W:R ratio	8 rounds for time:		None		3-5 mile run	75%-85% MHR	None	
		(a) Fan bike	15 calories						
		(b) Hand release push-up	× 10						

Five-Day Program, Phase 6

WEEK 2

	Day 1	Day 2	Day 3	Day 4	Day 5
(1)	High ankle hop — 2 × 10 (MR)	Broad jump — 1 × 3 (SR), 2 × 3 (MR)	Vertical jump — 1 × 5 (SR), 2 × 5 (MR)	High ankle hop — 2 × 10 (MR)	High ankle hop — 1 × 10 (MR)
(2)	Power skip — 2 × 4 each	Lateral bound — 1 × 4 each (SR), 2 × 4 each (MR)	50 yd shuttle with alt foot plant — × 6	Power skip — 2 × 4ea	Vertical jump — 1 × 5 (SR)
(3)	Bound — 1 × 4 each (SR), 2 × 4 each (MR)	MB scoop toss — 3 × 5	Hang clean low pull — 2 × 5, 4 × 3		Power skip — 2 × 4 each
(4) / (4a)	40 yd build-ups — × 6	Chin-up — 2 × 5, 4 × 8,6,6, 1 × AMRAP (>5 reps)	Inverted row — 1 × 5, 4 × 10		ACFT practice — 100% of previous ACFT results
(4b)		Lateral squat — 1 × 5 each, 4 × 5 each	Body saw — 4 × 10		
(5a)		Incline bench press — 2 × 5, 4 × 8,6,6	SA DB shoulder press — 1 × 5 each, 4 × 10 each		
(5b)		SB leg curl — 4 × 15	RFE DB SA split squat — 1 × 5 each, 4 × 10 each		
(6a)		Leg tuck — 4 × 5-20	RDL — 1 × 5, 3 × 5, 1 × 10		
(6b)		Facepull — 3 × 15	RG band pullapart — 4 × 15		
Conditioning	400 m repeats — × 9 at 5%-15% faster than 1-mile pace with 1:1 W:R ratio	8 rounds for time: (a) Fan bike — 15 calories (b) Hand release push-up — × 10	None	3-5 mile run — 75%-85% MHR	None

(continued)

Table 12.25 Five-Day Program, Phase 6 (continued)

WEEK 3

Day 1		Day 2		Day 3		Day 4		Day 5	
(1) High ankle hop	2 × 10 (MR)	(1) Broad jump	1 × 3 (SR) 2 × 3 (MR)	(1) Vertical jump	1 × 5 (SR) 2 × 5 (MR)	(1) High ankle hop	2 × 10 (MR)	(1) High ankle hop	1 × 10 (MR)
(2) Power skip	2 × 4 each	(2) Lateral bound	1 × 4 each (SR) 2 × 4 each (MR)	(2) 50 yd shuttle with alt foot plant	× 6	(2) Power skip	2 × 4 each	(2) Vertical jump	1 × 5 (SR)
(3) Bound	1 × 4 each (SR) 2 × 4 each (MR)	(3) MB scoop toss	3 × 5	(3) Hang clean low pull	2 × 5 3 × 3			(3) Power skip	2 × 4 each
(4) 40 yd build-ups	× 6	(4a) Chin-up	2 × 5 3 × 5	(4a) Inverted row	1 × 5 3 × 10			(4) ACFT practice	All-out
		(4b) Lateral squat	1 × 5 each 3 × 5 each	(4b) Body saw	4 × 10				
		(5a) Incline bench press	2 × 5 3 × 5	(5a) SA DB shoulder press	1 × 5 each 3 × 10 each				
		(5b) SB leg curl	4 × 10	(5b) RFE DB SA split squat	1 × 5 each 3 × 10 each				
		(6a) Leg tuck	4 × 5-20	(6a) RDL	1 × 5 3 × 5				
		(6b) Facepull	3 × 15	(6b) RG band pullapart	4 × 15				
Conditioning		**Conditioning**		**Conditioning**		**Conditioning**		**Conditioning**	
400 m repeats	× 9 at 5%-15% faster than 1-mile pace with 1:1 W:R ratio	8 rounds for time:		None		3-5 mile run	75%-85% MHR	None	
		(a) Fan bike	15 calories						
		(b) Hand release push-up	× 10						

Five-Day Program, Phase 6

WEEK 4

Day 1		Day 2		Day 3		Day 4		Day 5	
(1) High ankle hop	2 × 10 (MR)	(1) Broad jump	1 × 3 (SR) 2 × 3 (MR)	(1) Vertical jump	1 × 5 (SR) 2 × 5 (MR)	(1) High ankle hop	2 × 10 (MR)	(1) High ankle hop	1 × 10 (MR)
(2) Power skip	2 × 4 each	(2) Lateral bound	1 × 4 each (SR) 1 × 4 each (MR)	(2) 50 yd shuttle with alt foot plant	× 4	(2) Power skip	2 × 4 each	(2) Vertical jump	1 × 5 (SR)
(3) 40 yd build-ups	× 4	(3) MB scoop toss	3 × 5	(3) Hang clean low pull	2 × 5 3 × 3			(3) Power skip	2 × 4 each
		(4a) Chin-up	2 × 5 3 × 5	(4a) Inverted row	1 × 5 3 × 10			(4) ACFT practice	80% of last week's ACFT results
		(4b) Lateral squat	1 × 5 each 2 × 5 each	(4b) Body saw	3 × 10				
		(5a) Incline bench press	2 × 5 3 × 5	(5a) SA DB shoulder press	1 × 5 each 3 × 6 each				
		(5b) SB leg curl	2 × 15	(5b) RFE DB SA split squat	1 × 5 each 3 × 6 each				
		(6a) Leg tuck	2 × 5-20	(6a) RDL	1 × 5 3 × 5				
		(6b) Facepull	2 × 15	(6b) RG band pullapart	3 × 15				
Conditioning		**Conditioning**		**Conditioning**		**Conditioning**		**Conditioning**	
400 m repeats	× 5 at 5%-15% faster than 1-mile pace with 1:1 W:R ratio	**6 rounds for time:**		None		3-5 mile walk	No added weight	None	
		(a) Fan bike	15 calories						
		(b) Hand release push-up	× 10						

Workout and Exercise Descriptions

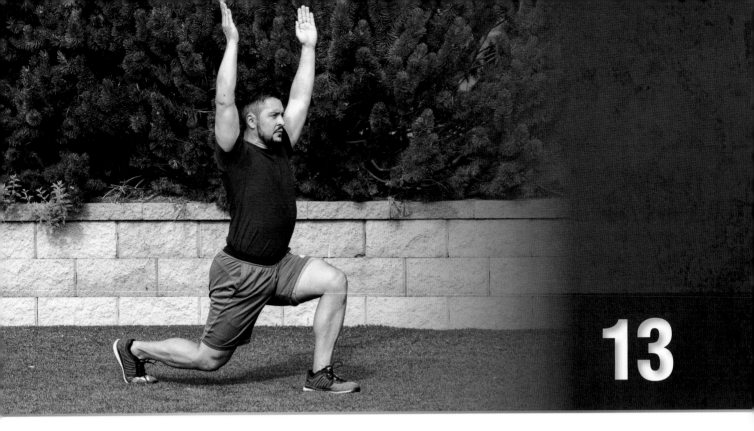

13

Warm-Up

Unfortunately, the benefits of a thorough, progressive, and specific warm-up routine are often sacrificed because of time constraints, impatience, or a lack of knowledge on how to design and implement an effective warm-up routine. A targeted warm-up maximizes the efforts of your training session while reducing the risk of injury. It also provides a safe and controlled setting to demonstrate and improve your movement competency by rehearsing common movement patterns at slower speeds and lighter loads. This chapter provides you with a general warm-up to incorporate before each day of training and lends advice for when you prefer to include additional or substitutive exercises.

Your warm-up should be progressive in nature. This means it should start general, slow, stable, and simple, and progress toward being specific, fast, less stable, and more complex. Consider learning marksmanship as an analogy. You start with learning the fundamentals in a static, stable position without ammunition, and ultimately progress to dynamically moving and shooting with live rounds in real-world scenarios.

Within a warm-up, it does not get more specific than performing the exercise itself. However, prior to warm-up sets on assigned exercises, you can incorporate components of the session to set the stage. These components target the same muscles, tendons, joints, and movement patterns that are trained within the session. To squat effectively and safely, for example, you need adequate range of motion in the ankles, hips, and upper back, complemented by adequate stability in the knees and lower back. A proper warm-up helps achieve the necessary range of motion and stability before external load enters into the equation. The following warm-up routine prepares you for training by not only increasing blood flow and range of motion, but perhaps most importantly enhancing your neuromuscular coordination. It purposely involves no equipment. The routine will initially take a little longer to complete, but with increased proficiency, you should be able to complete it within 10 minutes. If time does not allow, reduce the warm-up by cutting repetitions and distance in half, but do not eliminate it!

Warm-Up Exercises Finder

GENERAL WARM-UP EXERCISES

General warm-up exercises simply increase blood flow. They also help shift focus from the morning commute or weekend shenanigans to the training task. These exercises are performed at low amplitude and a jog-level pace as a way to simply get moving. In the absence of space, you can simply jog or lightly skip in place, adding in arm movements as desired.

JOG WITH BACKPEDAL
3 × 20 Yards (or Meters) (Out and Back)

As simple as it sounds, jog down and backpedal back. You can add in some lazy arm swings or circles.

SIDE SHUFFLE

20 Yards (or Meters) (Out and Back)

Shuffle laterally and somewhat lazily, being sure to not cross the feet. This introduces some light lateral movement that is not too taxing or technical. Arm swings across the body or overhead are appropriate additions.

CARIOCA

20 Yards (or Meters) (Out and Back)

Move laterally while crossing the trail leg over the lead leg and letting the body rotate naturally. Keeping in mind this is a general warm-up, do not aggressively lift the trail leg over the lead leg, and do not aggressively rotate the body (see figure 13.1). Again, move at the pace of a jog.

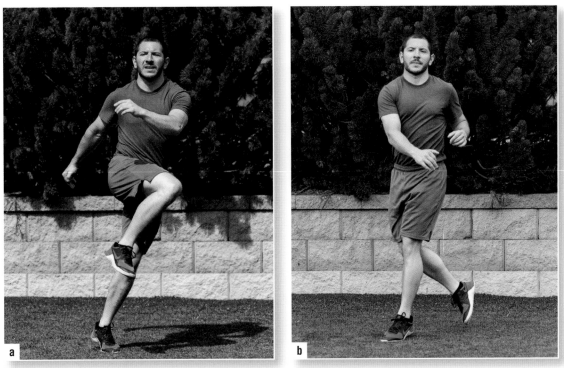

Figure 13.1   *(a)* Carioca with the leg crossed in front; *(b)* carioca with the leg crossed behind.

Another great general warm-up exercise for soldiers not prescribed within this program is jumping rope. A few hundred casually performed repetitions can provide a great general warm-up while challenging coordination in a safe way.

MOBILIZATION WARM-UP EXERCISES

Mobilization warm-up exercises aim to increase or preserve range of motion where soldiers are commonly restricted. While not an exhaustive list, soldiers are commonly restricted at the ankle, hip, upper back, and shoulder. These exercises are performed in a slow and controlled manner with a focus on pushing deliberately but not too aggressively into your end range. If time and equipment permit, you can precede these exercises with self-myofascial release (foam rolling) the muscles surrounding these joints.

STANDING ANKLE MOBILIZATION
10 Repetitions Each

With your hands placed against a wall, rack, or anything stationary, stagger your legs so the big toe of your lead foot is about 6 inches (15 cm) away from the wall and the toes of your trail leg are about 1 foot (30 cm) behind the heel of your lead leg. Keep your front foot flat on the floor, and drive your lead knee toward the wall to maximally dorsiflex your ankle. You may or may not feel a traditional stretch, but rest assured that you are mobilizing your ankle (see figure 13.2). Keep your trail leg relaxed.

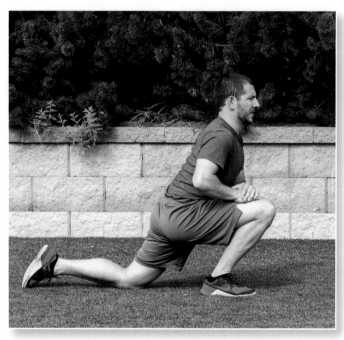

Figure 13.2   Standing ankle mobilization in a dorsiflexed position.

HALF-KNEELING HIP MOBILIZATION

10 Repetitions Each

Start in a half-kneeling position, forming a 90-degree angle at both knees and maintaining an upright torso. "Tuck your tail," by posteriorly tilt your pelvis. Squeeze the butt cheek on the leg that is down and shift your hips forward to elicit a slight stretch through the front of the hip on the leg that is down (see figure 13.3). Keep your abdominals tight to avoid arching excessively through your lower back.

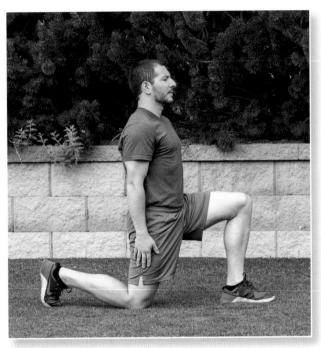

Figure 13.3   Half-kneeling hip mobilization in a stretched position.

TRI-PED UPPER BACK MOBILIZATION
10 Repetitions Each

From a kneeling position, sit back on your heels and post up on one hand while placing your other hand behind your head. Open up and rotate maximally through your upper back like you are trying to show your chest the ceiling, then diagonally crunch across your body by bringing your bent elbow behind your posted arm (see figure 13.4).

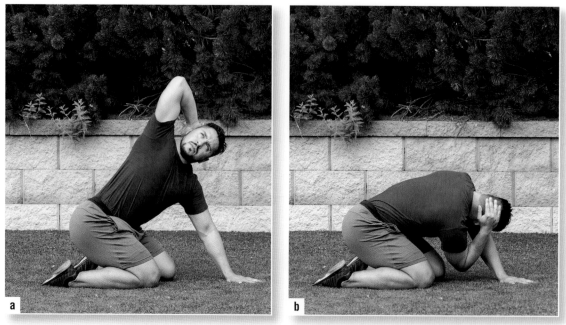

Figure 13.4 *(a)* Tri-ped upper back mobilization in an external rotation; *(b)* tri-ped upper back mobilization in an internal rotation.

WALL SHOULDER MOBILIZATION (WALL SLIDES)

10 Repetitions

Stand facing the wall with your toes a few inches away from it. With palms facing each other, place your arms and wrists against the wall with your arms at your sides, forming a W shape (*a*). Slowly slide your arms up the wall while straightening them until they are fully extended (*b*). Slowly return to the beginning position by sliding your arms back down the wall.

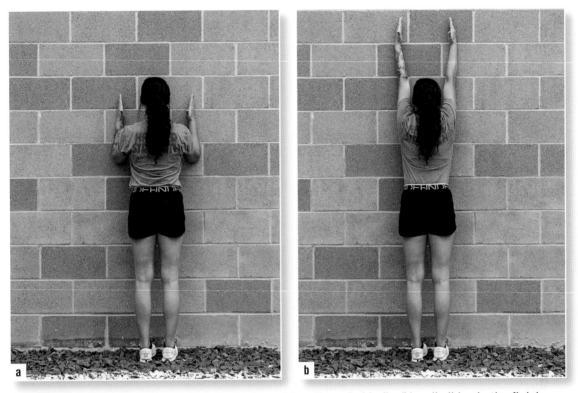

Figure 13.5   *(a)* Wall slides in the beginning position (from behind); *(b)* wall slides in the finish (overhead) position (from behind).

DYNAMIC WARM-UP EXERCISES

Dynamic warm-up exercises aim to move the body through full ranges of motion with an increased need for coordination. These are still performed in a controlled manner with an emphasis on proper positions and minimal movement compensations to achieve range of motion. Conveniently, these exercises can be performed in place or moving.

HAND WALK WITH YOGA PUSH-UP

5 Repetitions

Start from a tall standing position. Hinge your hips by sticking your butt back until your hands reach the ground, flexing minimally at the knees to feel a stretch down the back side of your body *(a)*. Actively engage the ground through your hands and walk them out until you are in the top of a push-up position *(b)*. Perform a full push-up and stick your butt in the air while pressing the ground overhead on the way up *(c)*. From there, walk your hands back toward your toes and then return to a tall standing position *(d)*.

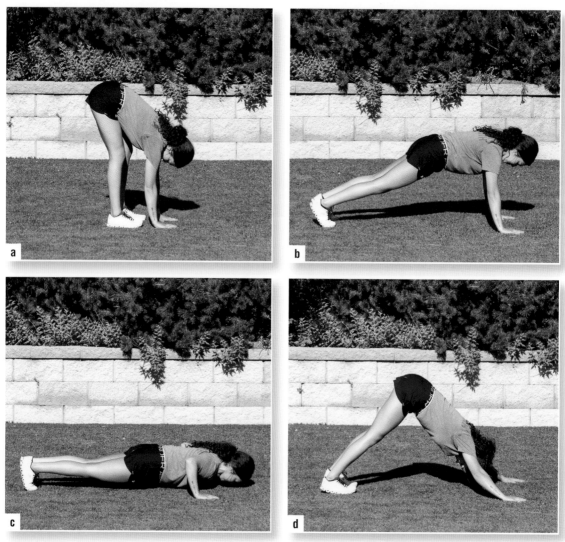

Figure 13.6   *(a)* Hand walk in the hinged position; *(b)* hand walk in a high plank position; *(c)* bottom of the yoga push-up position; *(d)* top of the yoga push-up position.

GROINER WITH ROTATION (WORLD'S GREATEST)

5 Repetitions Each

From the top of a push-up position, bring one foot to the outside of the same side's hand, placing it flat on the ground *(a)*. Arch your upper back and drive the back leg straight, then rotate the hand that is on the same side as the lead leg up toward the ceiling *(b)*. Return your hand back to the push-up position before bringing your leg back to where it started. Repeat for the opposite side of the body.

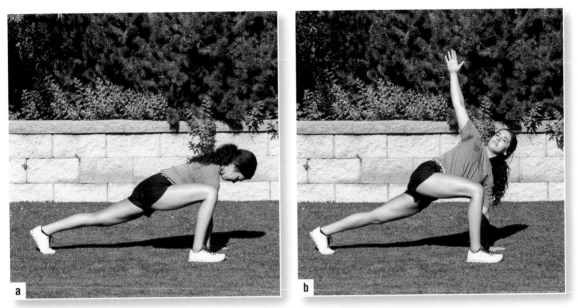

Figure 13.7   *(a)* Groiner position (without rotation); *(b)* groiner position (with rotation).

SQUAT TO STAND

10 Repetitions

Hinge your hips by sending your butt back in order to get your hands down, similar to the hand walk. Grab your feet under your toes while maintaining a stretch through your posterior. Keep your arms completely straight and your feet flat on the ground while continuously pulling up on your feet *(a)*. Drop your butt down and drive your knees outside your elbows while arching your back until you are holding a deep squat position. With your arms still straight, let go of your feet and raise your arms overhead to form a Y *(b)*. Maintain the Y and stand up.

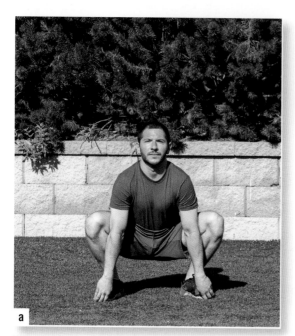 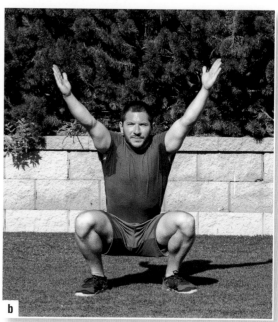

Figure 13.8   *(a)* Squat to stand in the bottom position with feet grab; *(b)* squat to stand in the bottom position with the arms up.

HIGH KNEE PULL

10 Repetitions Each

Stand tall on one leg while pulling the opposite knee to your chest. Keep your airborne ankle flexed so your toes are pointing toward the ceiling, and keep the chest held tall throughout the movement (see figure 13.9). Repeat on the opposite leg.

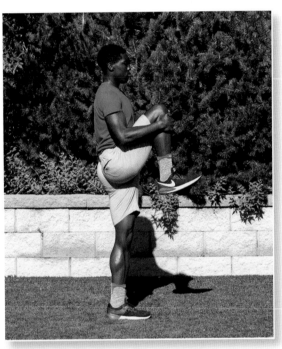

Figure 13.9   High knee pull in the top position (from the side).

QUAD WALK

10 Repetitions Each

Stand tall on one leg while bringing your opposite heel toward your butt. Grab the ankle of your lifted leg and continue to pull it toward your butt while staying tall through the torso (see figure 13.10). You can optionally reach toward the ceiling with your opposite arm. Repeat on the opposite leg.

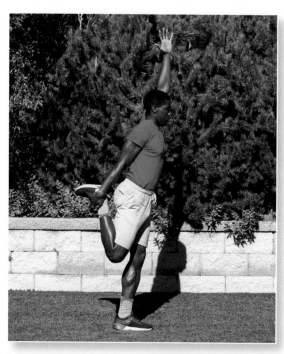

Figure 13.10   Quad walk in the top position (from the side).

LUNGE WITH ARMS OVERHEAD

10 Repetitions Each

Step back or travel forward by lunging while keeping your arms formed in a Y overhead. Both knees should be bent, with the lead one at a slightly acute angle and the rear one at a slightly obtuse angle. Staying tall through the torso and keeping the arms up, drive up through the lead leg to return to a standing position (see figure 13.11). Repeat on the opposite leg.

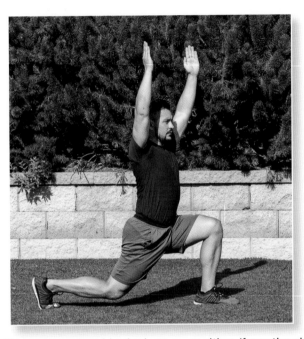

Figure 13.11   Lunge with arms overhead in the bottom position (from the side).

SINGLE-LEG ROMANIAN DEADLIFT

10 Repetitions Each

Stand on one leg, keeping a natural bend in the knee. Hinge your hips and drive the opposite leg backward while keeping a strong, straight line from your head through your heel until your body forms a T (see figure 13.12). Maintain level hips throughout the movement.

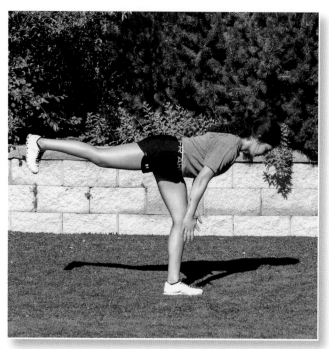

Figure 13.12   Single-leg Romanian deadlift in the hinged position (from the side).

LATERAL LUNGE

10 Repetitions Each

If performed in place, step wider than you think you want to while keeping both toes facing fairly straight forward *(a)*. Keep your feet flat while you sit back through your hips and flex the knee of the stepping leg; keep the trail leg straight *(b)*. Keep your knee inside of your ankle and your hip inside your knee to create an effective platform from which to push. Drive through your lead leg to return to your original standing position. Repeat on the opposite leg. If you find yourself moving, step slightly less far apart to start. Continue to shift your hips back, but let your knee and hip travel slightly ahead of your lead foot. Drive down and back through your lead leg, and bring your trail leg alongside it to finish in a standing position about one yard (1 m) ahead of where you started. Turn your body 180 degrees and continue forward progress on the opposite leg.

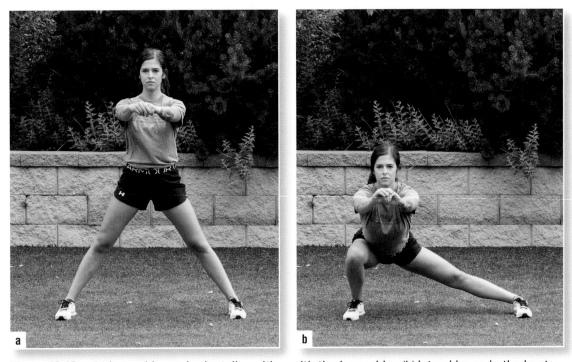

Figure 13.13   *(a)* Lateral lunge in the tall position with the legs wide; *(b)* lateral lunge in the bent-knee position (from the front).

MOVEMENT SKILL EXERCISES

It is no secret that traditional APFT training does not enhance general athleticism. Movement skill exercises are faster paced than dynamic warm-up exercises and help reinstate some athleticism into your movements. Where dynamic warm-up exercises involve a controlled range of motion, movement skill exercises involve momentum and take you through patterns occurring closer to "game speed."

HIGH KNEE MARCH
10 Yards (or Meters) or 10 Seconds

Stand tall, forming a straight line from your feet through the crown of your head. Maintain this tall stance through one leg while lifting the opposite knee to 90 degrees. Keep your forward elbow at 90 degrees with the arm opposite your lifted knee swinging forward and, simultaneously, your same side arm swinging back. Keep your hands relaxed with your lead hand at about chest height and your trail hand just past your pants pocket. Maintain a stretch through your lower leg by keeping your toes up throughout the march. Begin to march with opposite arms and legs moving in unison (see figure 13.14). Do not worry too much about forward progress.

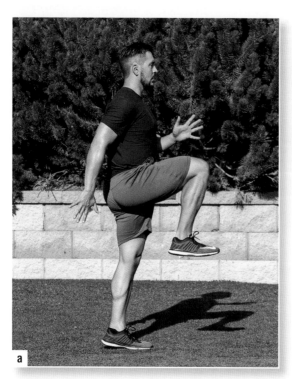 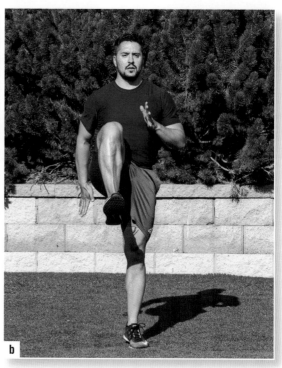

Figure 13.14   *(a)* High knee march (from the side); *(b)* high knee march (from the front).

HIGH KNEE SKIP

10 Yards (or Meters) or 10 Seconds

The skip includes the exact same pattern as the march with only one exception. Instead of making a single foot contact with the ground each step, your foot will punch the ground and make you float briefly before landing again on the same foot, immediately followed by the opposite leg punching the ground (see figure 13.15). The skip requires more coordination than the march. Sometimes starting with your hands on your head or holding a light object overhead helps you focus on the legs and not worry so much about coordinating the arm movements.

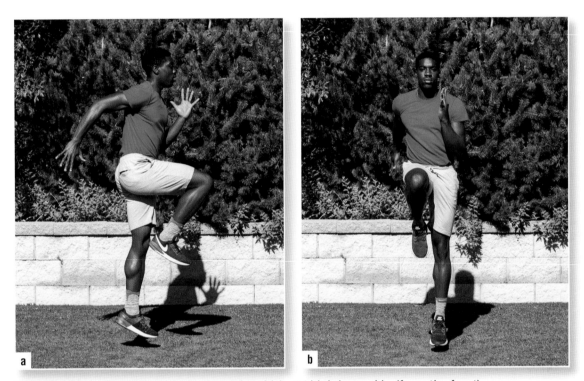

Figure 13.15   *(a)* High knee skip (from the side); *(b)* high knee skip (from the front).

HIGH KNEES

10 Yards (or Meters) or 10 Seconds

High knees are a fast version of the march. Your goal is to churn your legs over as fast as possible while maintaining a tall posture. Achieve as many foot contacts as possible within the distance or time specified.

LATERAL SHUFFLE
10 Yards (or Meters) Each

Begin in an athletic stance. Your feet should be wider than your knees, and your knees wider than your hips. Sit back while keeping your chest up, and hold your arms as if waiting to catch a ball. Your weight should be on the balls of your feet, and you should feel like you can move easily and quickly in any direction *(a)*. To move laterally, push off the inside of the trail leg and keep your lead leg out in front of you, staying low throughout *(b)*. To stop, brake through the inside of your lead foot and finish in the same athletic stance in which you started *(c-d)*. Avoid clapping your feet underneath you, getting tall, or letting your center of mass hover over your lead foot. These common faults can result in tripping, difficulty changing direction, and even ankle injuries. Perform one set in each direction with a pause on each shuffle, and a second set moving fluidly to cover the distance.

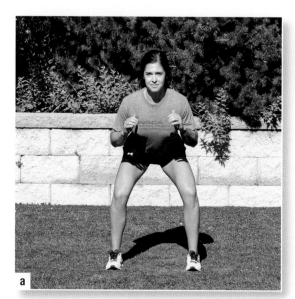 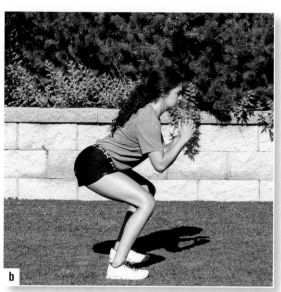

Figure 13.16 *(a-b)* Athletic stance (front and side view).

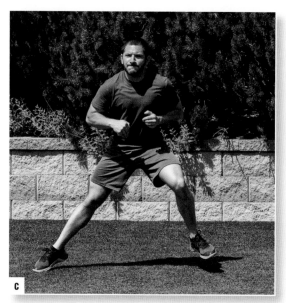 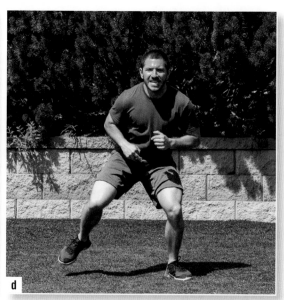

Figure 13.16 *(c)* Lateral shuffle (lead leg is bent and hovering, and the trail leg is extended); *(d)* lateral shuffle (change of direction moment).

ACCELERATION AND DECELERATION
4 Repetitions

Start in a staggered stance position with one arm and the opposite leg forward. Push through both legs to initiate a sprint. At the 10-yard (9 m) mark, drop your hips and shorten your steps to decelerate as quickly as possible, coming to a dead stop in an athletic stance. Walk back to the start and repeat with your opposite leg forward in your staggered stance.

NEURAL ACTIVATION EXERCISES

Neural activation exercises wake up your central nervous system by moving your body as fast as possible over a short period of time while also challenging your coordination. They are a great final warm-up before performing explosive movements such as plyometrics and sprints.

BENT-KNEE RUN
5 Seconds

Begin in an athletic stance, as described within the lateral shuffle. Maintaining the integrity of your stance, run in place as fast as possible. Your feet will make a machine gun sound against the floor. To make the exercise more challenging, slowly alternate your arms as you do when running in place.

BENT-KNEE LATERAL POGO
5 Seconds

This is performed similar to the bent-knee run, except you should pick your feet up and put them down at the same time, moving laterally back and forth a few inches at a time.

BENT-KNEE ROTATIONS

5 Seconds

Start in an athletic stance. Counterrotate your upper and lower body in a fast hopping motion so that your feet land at 45-degree angles to the left and right while your torso faces straight ahead throughout the exercise (see figure 13.17).

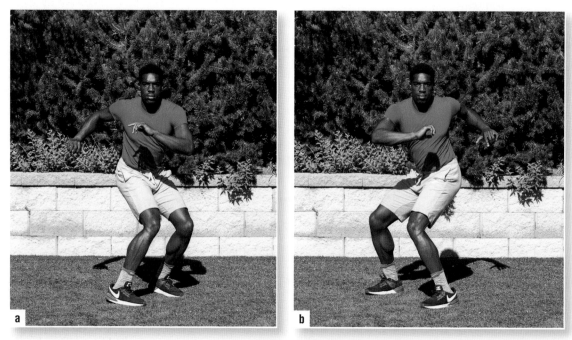

Figure 13.17   *(a)* Bent-knee rotation (left); *(b)* bent-knee rotation (right).

SPECIFIC WARM-UP EXERCISES

Specific warm-up exercises involve performing lighter versions of the exercises within your program or the same movement in a different way. An example of the former would be an empty barbell bench press. An example of the latter would be a band pulldown before a set of pull-ups. Specific warm-ups help you maximize the effectiveness of your working sets and should not be counted. Sometimes the program within this book includes specific warm-up exercises, but you are welcome to include them wherever you see fit.

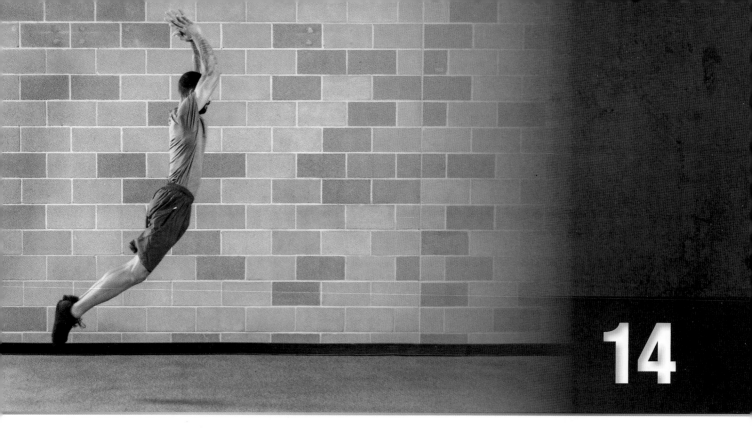

Power Exercises

14

Power exercises, which are characterized by **triple extension**, emphasize the expression of power due to a high rate of force development through the ankles, knees, and hips. The goal of these exercises is to maximize force output while minimizing the time it takes to produce that force. These exercises contribute directly to the SPT and SDC but also strongly support the 2MR. Most of these exercises do not require equipment, and those that do can easily be substituted with those that do not.

ALTERNATIVE POWER EXERCISES

The power exercises included in the chapter 12 programs are the most preferred exercises because they relate to the ACFT. If you do not have the needed equipment to do a preferred exercise, you will need to choose an alternative exercise. Go to table 14.1 and find the exercise you need to replace along the top row; the name will not include the piece of equipment. Next, find the equipment options to which you have access in the left column. Your alternative exercise options are where the column of the exercise you are replacing intersects the rows of the types of equipment you have access to. Choose the option that best mimics the position, movement, and resistance level of the preferred exercise in the chapter 12 programs. It is important to note that not every type of equipment supports an alternative exercise, but at least a bodyweight replacement exists for every exercise, so there is no excuse to entirely omit a programmed exercise.

Power Exercises Finder

Table 14.1 Alternative Power Exercises

	Vertical jump	Broad jump	Squat jump	Quarter squat jump	Tuck jump	High ankle hop	Power skip	Bound	Lateral bound	Medicine ball scoop toss	Hang clean low pull
Trap bar			↑	↑						↑	↑
Barbell											
Dumbbell											
Kettlebell			Squat jump	Quarter squat jump						Squat jump	Hang clean low pull
Sandbag											
Band											
Suspension trainer			↓	↓						↓	↓
Body weight	Vertical jump	Broad jump	Squat jump	Quarter squat jump	Tuck jump	High ankle hop	Power skip	Bound	Lateral bound	Vertical jump	Vertical jump

VERTICAL JUMP

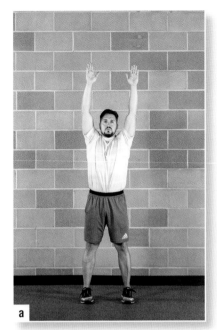
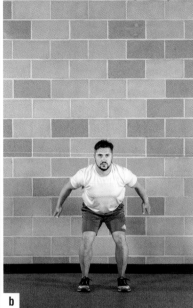
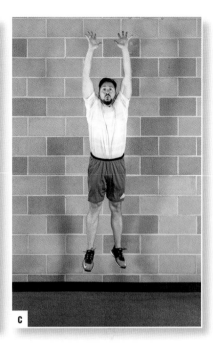

SETUP

Stand with the feet hip-width apart and clear of any obstacles.

EXECUTION

1. Maintain a rigid spine—neutral to slightly arched (not rounded)—throughout this entire movement.

2. Raise your hands over your head to allow for a more forceful descent *(a)*.

3. Throw your hands down as you shift your hips backward, allowing your hips and knees to flex slightly.

4. This forceful descent should cease once you reach a comfortable end position, with your shoulders above your hips, and your hips above your knees *(b)*. Instantly reverse.

5. Drive your whole foot into the ground while extending the hips, knees, and then ankles, and simultaneously throw your arms upward. This forceful event should launch your entire body into the air *(c)*.

6. Once gravity takes over, prepare to contact the ground with the intent of allowing the ankle, knees, and hips to flex once the feet touch the ground. Shift the hips backward and allow the arms to move down and back as well.

7. Once the feet touch the ground, return to step 2 and continue for the prescribed number of repetitions.

COMMON FAULTS

■ *Knees caving in.* Focus on maintaining the knees' alignment with the feet. Thinking about pushing the knees outward on the way down and up can assist with this.

■ *Not using the arms.* Reexamine the effort to use the arms to create force both on the descent and the jump portion of the movement. This will assist with a high jump and full hip extension.

SQUAT JUMP

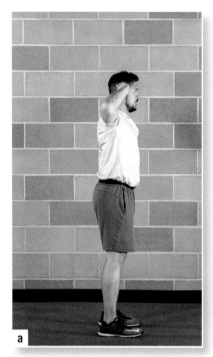
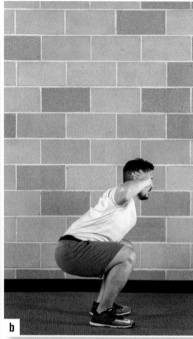
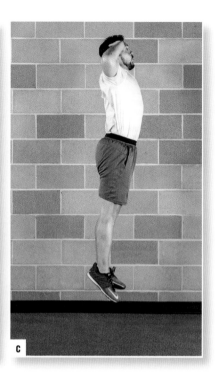

SETUP

1. Place your hands on your head, allowing the elbows to point out to the side.

2. Feet should be aligned at shoulder width or slightly wider.

3. Feet should be angled anywhere from neutral (straight ahead) to turned out at a 30-degree angle.

4. Maintain a neutral spine position.

5. Keep whole-foot pressure: The feet should be flat on the floor with obvious pressure driving through the heels, balls of the feet, and big toes.

VARIATION SETUP

1. If holding dumbbells, kettlebells, or a trap bar, keep your arms straight at your side (or goblet style, against your chest with two hands, if it is a single dumbbell or kettlebell).

2. If loading with a barbell or sandbag, keep it tight to your upper back and shoulders as in a squat.

3. If loading with a band, wrap it under the center of your feet, over your shoulders, and behind your neck *(d)*.

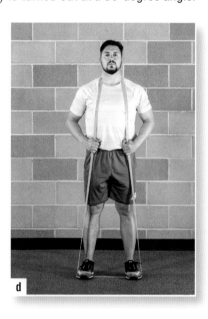

EXECUTION

1. Brace or create tension in the torso in preparation to support the weight and maintain a neutral spine position *(a)*.

2. As fast as you while maintaining control, descend downward by simultaneously flexing the knees and hips.

3. The knees track in line with your feet; do not let them cave in.

4. The feet remain flat on the floor with whole-foot pressure during the descent.

5. Go as low as you can while maintaining the integrity of the lumbar curve or a neutral spine, as well as proper ankle, knee, and hip alignment *(b)*.

6. As soon as you hit your lowest position, instantly drive your feet into the floor as forcefully as you can, forcing your body upward.

7. Continue to extend forcefully until your hips and knees are fully extended, forcing additional effort to transfer from your ankle through the balls of your feet, launching your body into the air *(c)*.

8. Once gravity takes over, prepare to contact the floor with the intent of allowing the ankle, knees, and hips to flex once the feet touch the floor.

9. Once the feet touch the floor, return to step 2 and continue for the prescribed number of repetitions.

VARIATION EXECUTION

1. Added load should not compromise body position during any part of the exercise.

2. Keep the arms straight if holding a load, and keep them tight to the body if rear loaded.

COMMON FAULTS

■ *Not going low enough.* Have someone watch you from the side to make sure you are at least going low enough to have your hips in line and parallel to the floor. If you cannot at least go that low while maintaining a neutral spine, be more conscious of the effort to drive your knees out throughout the entire movement. If that heightened consciousness does not correct the issue, you should only go as low as you can while maintaining that neutral position.

■ *Knees caving in.* Reexamine the effort to maintain the knees' alignment with the feet. Thinking about pushing the knees outward on the way down and the way up can assist with this.

QUARTER SQUAT JUMP

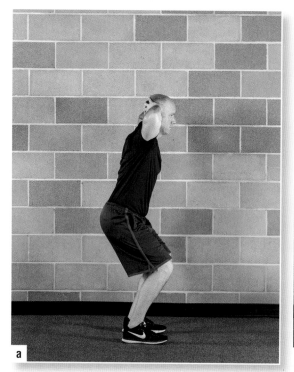

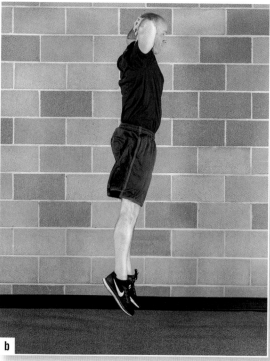

SETUP

1. Place your hands behind your head as if you are a prisoner.

2. The feet should be hip- to shoulder-width apart and aligned in a neutral or slightly turned-out position.

VARIATION SETUP

1. If holding dumbbells, kettlebells, or a trap bar, keep your arms straight at your side (or goblet style, against your chest with two hands, if it is a single dumbbell or kettlebell).

2. If loading with a barbell or sandbag, keep it tight to your upper back and shoulders as in a squat.

3. If loading with a band, wrap it under the center of your feet, over your shoulders, and behind your neck *(c)*.

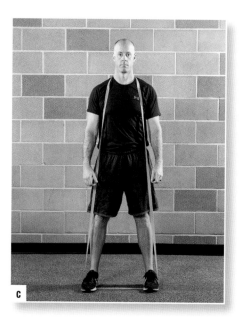

EXECUTION

1. Brace or create tension in the torso in preparation to support the weight and maintain a rigid spine—neutral to slightly arched (not rounded)—throughout this entire movement.
2. As fast as you can while maintaining control, descend downward by simultaneously flexing the knees and hips.
3. The hips should shift slightly backward, and the knees track in line with your feet; do not let them cave inward.
4. The knees should only flex about 45 degrees from the vertical position *(a)*.
5. The feet remain flat on the floor with whole-foot pressure during the descent.
6. Once you hit the bottom position, instantly drive your feet into the ground as forcefully as you can, forcing your body upward.
7. Continue to extend forcefully until your hips, knees, and then ankles are fully extended, forcing the upward momentum created to launch your body into the air *(b)*.
8. Once gravity takes over, prepare to contact the ground with the intent of allowing the ankle, knees, and hips to flex once the feet touch the ground.
9. Once the feet touch the ground, return to step 1 and continue for the prescribed number of repetitions.

VARIATION EXECUTION

1. Added load should not compromise body position during any part of the exercise.
2. Keep the arms straight if holding a load, and keep them tight to the body if rear loaded.

COMMON FAULT

■ *Knees caving in.* Focus on maintaining the knees' alignment with the feet. Thinking about pushing the knees outward on the way down and the way up can assist with this.

BROAD JUMP

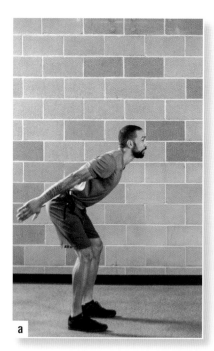 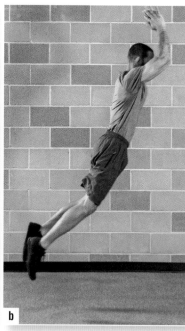 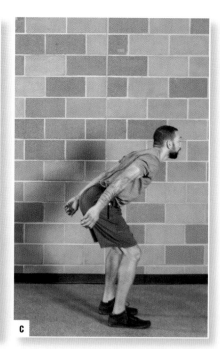

SETUP

Stand with feet hip-width apart.

EXECUTION

1. Maintain a rigid spine—neutral to slightly arched (not rounded)—throughout this entire movement.

2. Raise your hands over your head to allow for a more forceful descent.

3. Throw your hands down as you shift your hips backward, allowing your hips and knees to flex slightly *(a)*.

4. This forceful descent should cease once you reach the lowest comfortable position you can reverse without hesitation.

5. Drive your feet into the ground while extending the hips, knees, and then ankles, and simultaneously throw your arms up and forward. This forceful event should launch your entire body into the air at about a 45-degree angle to the floor *(b)*.

6. Once gravity takes over, prepare to contact the ground with the intent of allowing the ankle, knees, and hips to flex once the feet touch the ground, to absorb the force created by your forward movement and downward projection *(c)*.

7. Once the feet touch the ground, return to step 2 and continue for the prescribed number of repetitions.

COMMON FAULTS

- *Knees caving in.* Focus on maintaining the knees' alignment with the feet. Thinking about pushing the knees outward on the way down and the way up can assist with this.

- *Not using the arms.* Reexamine the effort to use the arms to create force both on the descent and the jump portion of the movement. This will assist with a high jump and full hip extension.

- *Throwing the arms backward as you jump forward.* Concentrate on projecting every part of your body in the intended direction of movement.

TUCK JUMP

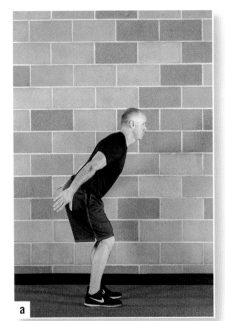 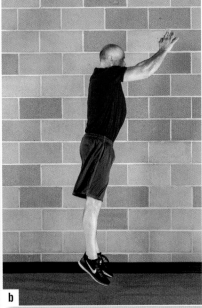 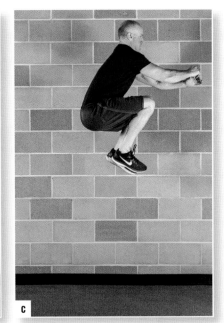

SETUP

Stand with the feet hip-width apart and clear of any obstacles *(a)*.

EXECUTION

1. Maintain a rigid spine—neutral to slightly arched (not rounded)—throughout this entire movement.
2. Drive your feet into the ground while extending the hips, knees, and then ankles, and simultaneously drive your arms upward. This forceful event should launch your entire body into the air *(b)*.
3. As you launch yourself into the air, bring your knees up to a point where your thighs are parallel to the floor *(c)*.
4. Once gravity takes over, prepare to contact the ground with the intent of allowing the ankle, knees, and hips to flex once the feet touch the ground, preparing instantly for the next jump.
5. Once the feet touch the ground, return to step 2 and continue for the prescribed number of repetitions.

COMMON FAULTS

- *Knees caving in.* Focus on maintaining the knees' alignment with the feet.
- *Taking too much time on the ground.* The intent of this movement is to anticipate the ground contact and launch yourself back into the air as soon and as high as possible without any hesitation on the ground.

HIGH ANKLE HOP

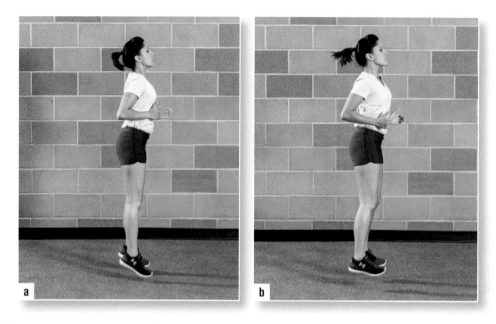

SETUP

1. Stand with the feet hip-width apart and clear of any obstacles.
2. The elbows should be fixed at a 90-degree angle positioned behind your torso in a cocked and ready position.

EXECUTION

1. Maintain a rigid spine—neutral to slightly arched (not rounded)—throughout this entire movement.
2. The legs should remain relatively straight during the movement *(a)*.
3. Keeping the elbows at about a 90-degree angle, drive the arms forward and upward until the hands are at about shoulder height, simultaneously driving the balls of your feet into the ground and extending your ankles to launch your body into the air. The arms should stop once the hands are at shoulder height, to assist in the elevation of your body and, in turn, jump height. (NOTE: These arm and foot positions were not quite captured in photo *(b)*, but they are important aspects of the exercise.)
4. Once gravity takes over, prepare to contact the ground with the intent of driving the balls of your feet into the ground instantly.
5. Drive the balls of your feet into the ground while simultaneously repeating the aggressive arm action to launch your body back into the air with the least amount of time spent on the ground as possible and getting as high as possible.

COMMON FAULTS

■ *Taking too much time on the ground between repetitions.* This reduces the elastic training effect intended. Do not react to the contact of the ground; anticipate it. Anticipate the contact, force, and speed needed to instantly reverse your downward descent. It is about timing.

■ *Not using your arms.* Once you get comfortable with the lower-body portion of this exercise, incorporate the arms. You will not get the full training effect without their assistance.

POWER SKIP

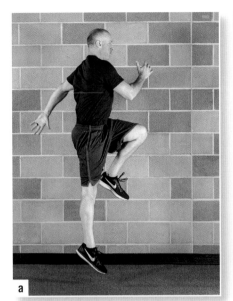
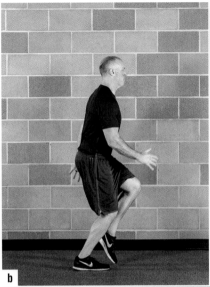
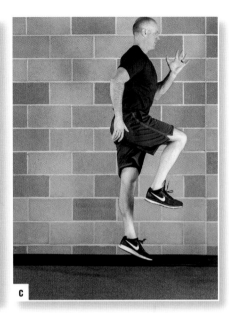

SETUP

Start by walking or taking a few slow jog-like steps forward as you prepare to engage in this action of skipping.

EXECUTION

1. Maintain a rigid spine—neutral to slightly arched (not rounded)—throughout this entire movement.

2. Initiate the act of the bound by driving your down leg's foot into the ground to propel your body up and forward.

3. As you drive your down leg's foot into the ground, you should simultaneously punch your front leg's knee up and forward until the thigh is parallel to the ground *(a)*.

4. As you punch the knee forward, allow your arms to move in a running-like fashion (e.g., left knee forward, right arm forward).

5. The forward arm should near 90 degrees of flexion as it swings forward, stopping abruptly when the hand is at shoulder height.

6. Upon returning to the ground, the roles of each leg and arm switch *(b)*.

7. As the down leg's foot contacts the ground, a short skipping step occurs in preparation for the next up and forward propulsion *(c)*; each repetition will contain two ground contacts per feet.

8. Upon the second contact of the down leg, the process repeats itself starting with step 2.

COMMON FAULT

- *Not moving forward far enough.* Try to focus on projecting your body up and forward at about a 45-degree angle to the ground. Try to float in the air as long as possible.

BOUND

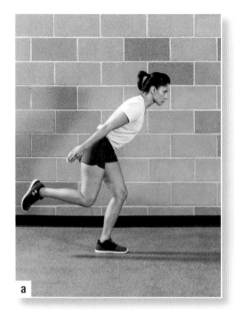
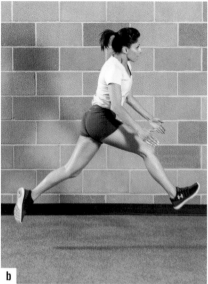
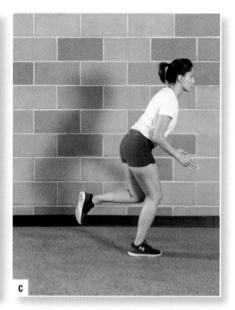

SETUP

Start by walking or taking a few slow jog-like steps forward as you prepare to engage in this action of bounding.

EXECUTION

1. Maintain a rigid spine—neutral to slightly arched (not rounded)—throughout this entire movement.

2. Initiate the act of the bound by driving your down leg's foot into the ground to propel your body forward and slightly upward *(a)*.

3. As you drive your down leg's foot into the ground, you should simultaneously punch your front leg's knee up and forward until the thigh is nearly parallel to the ground *(b)*.

4. As you punch the knee forward, use your arms to assist in creating forward and upward momentum.

5. The arms should near 90 degrees of flexion as they swing forward, stopping abruptly when the hands are at shoulder height.

6. The combination of these three simultaneous actions should be executed with the intent of floating in the air as long as possible before having to repeat the action when the legs switch roles after landing on the ground on one foot *(c)*.

COMMON FAULTS

- *Turning it into a skip.* Each foot should only contact the ground once before transitioning to the other foot.

- *Turning it into a run.* Make sure that there is some upward propulsion as well, allowing you to float between contacts. Exaggerate the upward effort a little more.

LATERAL BOUND

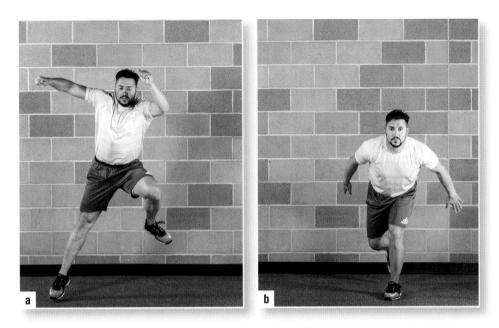

SETUP

Start in a semi-squat position, with the foot of the leg on the side you are going to jump toward slightly elevated from the ground.

EXECUTION

1. Maintain a rigid spine—neutral to slightly arched (not rounded)—throughout this entire movement.

2. Initiate the act of the bound by driving your down leg's foot, with an emphasis on the pressure driving through the inside ball of the foot, into the ground to propel your body up and laterally.

3. The inside leg should perform a lateral and upward swing, punching the knee to assist in creating momentum.

4. As you drive your foot into the ground and punch your inside knee up and laterally, use your arms to execute a lateral swing in the direction you are jumping, to assist in the propulsion *(a)*.

5. The combination of these three simultaneous actions should be executed with the intent of floating in the air as long as possible before having to repeat the action in the opposite direction when the legs switch roles after you land on the ground on one foot *(b)*.

COMMON FAULT

- *Falling from side to side, instead of bounding.* Focus on propelling your body up and laterally, not just laterally. Also, reexamine the intent to get as high as possible while also going as far as possible, which is typically accomplished by a 45-degree propulsion from the ground.

MEDICINE BALL SCOOP TOSS

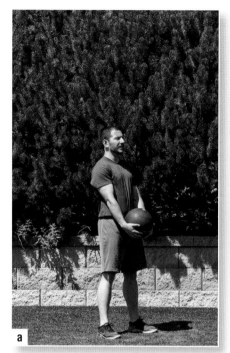
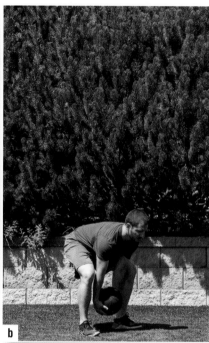
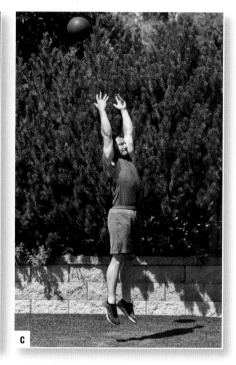

SETUP

1. Make sure no overhead obstacles exist.

2. The feet should be shoulder-width apart (or wide enough for the medicine ball to fit between your legs) and aligned in a neutral position or turned slightly outward.

3. The medicine ball should be held in front of the body at arm's length, as if it were hanging toward the ground *(a)*.

4. The hands should be placed on the sides and slightly under the ball in a comfortable position from which you can throw the ball.

EXECUTION

1. Maintain a rigid spine—neutral to slightly arched (not rounded)—throughout this entire movement.

2. Shift your hips backward, allowing your hips to flex, and simultaneously flex your knees slightly to allow the ball to lower between your legs toward the ground *(b)*. Descend as quickly as you can while maintaining control, then reverse the movement.

3. This rapid descent should cease once you reach a comfortable position, with your shoulders above your hips and your hips above your knees.

4. Once you reach this position, drive your feet into the ground, forcing the hips, knees, and then ankles to rapidly extend.

5. As the hips, knees, and then ankles rapidly extend, your torso and therefore the ball will move upward away from the ground. The ball should still be at arm's length away from the body.

6. Once you hit full extension of those joints, allow the momentum created to continue upward through your arms into the ball, releasing the ball at the highest point where you cannot put any more force into it *(c)*.

7. The momentum created will cause you to leave the ground as well *(c)*.

8. Once the ball is midair, be cautious as gravity begins to take over, making sure the ball does not hit you.

9. Do not try to catch the ball; allow it to hit the ground.

COMMON FAULT

- *Not shifting the hips backward on the initial descent.* Focus on shifting the hips backward. Although simply flexing the knees may make it easier to hold in the bottom position or allow you to see overhead, it reduces the hip involvement and therefore the amount of force it can produce, thereby reducing the value of the exercise.

ALTERNATIVE

The vertical jump is a simple alternative to this exercise.

HANG CLEAN LOW PULL

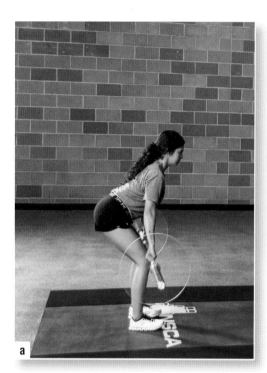 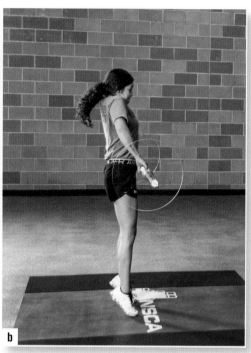

SETUP

1. With an overhand grip, grab the barbell so each hand is about a thumb's length from the smooth portion of the bar. The hands should be on the knurling and slightly outside of your thighs.

2. The bar should be touching your thighs but not resting on them.

3. The feet should be hip- to shoulder-width apart in a neutral to slightly turned-out position.

4. With a slight flex in your knees, push your hips backward, allowing your hips to flex as the bar travels downward on your thighs. Keep your arms straight the entire time.

5. Your back should remain in a neutral to slightly arched (not rounded) position throughout the movement.

6. Stop the descent once the bar is slightly higher than your knees *(a)*.

7. The feet should be flat on the floor with whole-foot pressure.

VARIATION SETUP

Dumbbells or a sandbag could be held in a similar fashion to a barbell, while kettlebells or a trap bar should be held with long arms.

EXECUTION

1. Keeping the torso rigid and the arms long, drive your feet into the floor, forcefully causing your hips, knees, and then ankles to extend.

2. Your back should remain in a neutral to slightly arched (not rounded) position throughout the movement.

3. The bar should travel as close as possible to your thigh without any friction that would increase resistance, causing it to slow down.

4. Once the hips, knees, and then the ankles are fully extended, forcefully shrug the shoulders straight up to continue the bar on its path *(b)*.

5. If you execute this in such a manner that results in you leaving the floor, be cautious on the landing, and consider adding a little more weight. It is still a good repetition, though.

6. Once fully extended and shrugged, gravity will quickly take over.

7. Anticipating the need to decelerate your body weight as well as the weight bar, prepare to slightly shift your hips backward and flex your knees once the descent begins.

8. Once the weight has ceased its descent, follow the initial setup procedure and execute again for the number of prescribed repetitions.

VARIATION EXECUTION

Variations should be executed the same with the exception of the position of the load changing as described in setup.

COMMON FAULT

■ *Not shifting hips backward on initial descent.* Focus on shifting the hips backward. Although simply flexing the knees may make it easier to hold the bar in the bottom position, it reduces the hip involvement and therefore the amount of force it can produce, thereby reducing the value of the exercise.

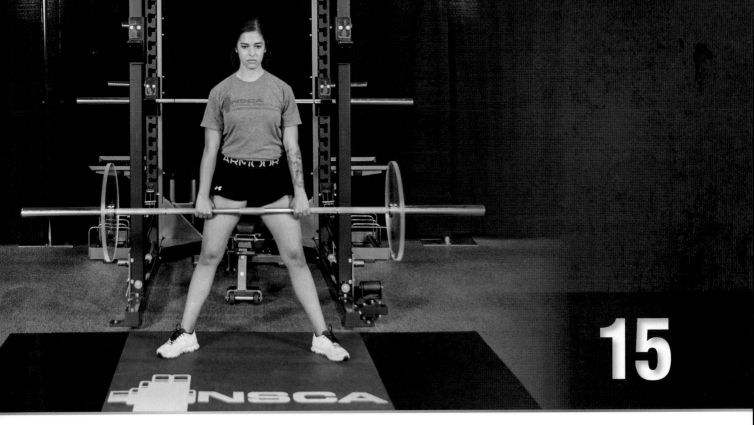

15

Lower Body Pulling Exercises

The lower body pulling exercises transfer directly to the MDL and also have potential to positively affect performance on the SPT, LTK, SDC, and 2MR). The deadlift and RDL exercises build leg, back, and grip strength, while more hamstring-intensive exercises such as the leg curl, glute-ham raise, and hip bridge build muscular strength and endurance of the lower body's posterior muscles. Keep in mind that for deadlifts and RDLs, nonconventional pieces of equipment such as tires and kegs as substitutes for resistance are not appropriate for all soldiers because picking up odd pieces of equipment is a skill in itself and requires an ability to maintain correct body position. Therefore, programmed exercises and their suggested alternatives typically use commonly available equipment such as barbells, kettlebells, dumbbells, suspension trainers, resistance bands, sandbags, and body weight.

Lower Body Pulling Exercises Finder

ALTERNATIVE LOWER BODY PULLING EXERCISES

The lower body pulling exercises included in the chapter 12 programs are the preferred exercises as they relate to the ACFT. If you do not have the needed equipment to do a preferred exercise, you will need to choose an alternative exercise. Go to table 15.1 and find the exercise you need to replace along the top row; the name will not include the piece of equipment. Next, find the equipment options you have access to along the left column. Your alternative exercise options are where the column of the exercise you are replacing intersects the rows of the types of equipment to which you have access. Choose the option that best mimics the position, movement, and resistance level of the preferred exercise in the chapter 12 programs. Note that not every type of equipment supports an alternative exercise, but at least a bodyweight replacement exists for every exercise, so there is no excuse to entirely omit a programmed exercise.

Table 15.1 Alternative Lower Body Pulling Exercises

	Deadlift	Sumo deadlift	Trap bar deadlift	RDL	Single-leg RDL	Stability ball leg curl	Glute-ham raise	Poor man's glute-ham raise	Hip bridge
Trap bar	↑	Deadlift	↑	↑	↑				
Barbell		↑							
Dumbbell									
Kettlebell	Deadlift	Sumo deadlift	Deadlift	RDL	Single-leg RDL				
Sandbag									
Band	↓	↓	↓	↓	↓				
Suspension trainer	↑	↑	↑	↑	↑	Leg curl	Leg curl	Leg curl	Hip bridge
Body weight	Single-leg squat ↓	Single-leg squat ↓	Single-leg squat ↓	Hip bridge ↓	Single-leg hip bridge ↓	Poor man's glute-ham raise	Poor man's glute-ham raise	Poor man's glute-ham raise	Hip bridge

POOR MAN'S GLUTE-HAM RAISE

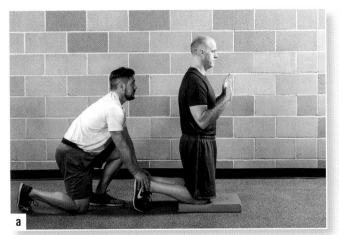 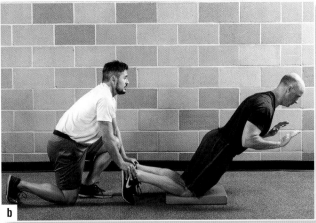

SETUP

1. Kneel on the ground on a foam pad or something soft to prevent discomfort for your knees as you perform the exercise.

2. Secure your feet under a roller pad attached to a rack or a stable and padded barbell, or have a partner hold your feet to the ground.

3. Once your feet are secured as close to the ground as possible, extend your hips so that your thighs and torso are aligned and perpendicular to the ground.

4. Bend your elbows and place your hands at chest height and as close to your torso as possible *(a)*. This is to help catch you, if needed.

EXECUTION

1. Keeping your hips engaged so that your thighs and torso stay in a straight line, allow your body to move forward and then downward, pushing yourself away from the pad or partner, allowing the knees to extend *(b)*.

2. Evenly control the descent so that it takes about three to four seconds to make your way all the way to the ground.

3. Once you touch the ground, drive your heels into the roller pad or partner and contract your hamstrings to pull your body back to the beginning position by flexing the knees.

4. Your torso and thighs should stay aligned the entire time.

5. It is OK to use a little push off the ground with your hands to get yourself started. The goal is to limit or remove this need over time, but it is rare that it is not necessary when starting out.

COMMON FAULTS

▪ *Starting the movement by flexing the hips.* Reexamine the intent to push hips into the pad as if pushing yourself away from the machine.

▪ *Initiating the return to the beginning position by flexing your knees first.* Focus on keeping the torso and thighs aligned the entire time, but if your hips flex to make the movement easier you should just use a little more of a push off from the ground until your strength increases.

DEADLIFT

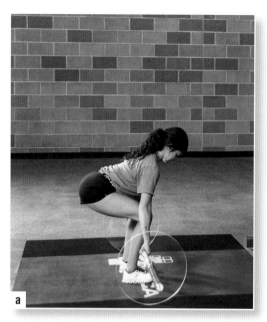
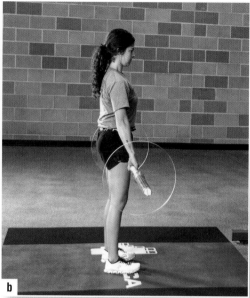

SETUP

1. The feet are hip- to shoulder-width apart and can be straight ahead or turned out to a 15-degree angle.

2. The bar is over the feet about 1 inch (3 cm) from the shins.

3. The grip width is slightly wider than hip width, allowing the arms to be straight and aligned outside the knees.

4. Using the bar to leverage yourself down, get into the bottom (beginning) position *(a)*.

    □ Keep the shoulders over the bar.

    □ Hip position is dependent on your build, but the hips are generally higher than your knees and below your shoulders.

    □ Maintain a neutral to slightly arched (not rounded) spine.

    □ The bar is still over the foot and almost touching your shins.

    □ Keep your feet flat on the floor.

VARIATION SETUP

1. Kettlebells, dumbbells, and sandbags will require grip width adjustment and possibly a deeper bottom position because their handles are lower to the floor. The bottom position should not compromise the integrity of a neutral spine, so raise the "floor" as needed to be able to safely use these pieces of equipment. A single kettlebell, dumbbell, or sandbag will be placed directly between your feet *(c)* while two of each will be placed outside your feet; this might require a slightly narrower stance.

2. If using a band, it will loop under the feet with the remainder of the setup unchanged. Adjust where you grip the band to determine the amount of resistance, keeping in mind it will be greatest at the top or lockout position.

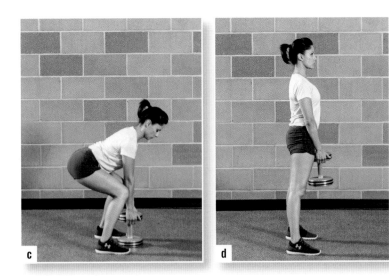

EXECUTION

1. Take the slack out of the bar by tightening the lats and putting pressure into the floor with your feet. To take the slack out of the bar, use the bar to lower yourself down into the beginning position, creating full-body tension. You should hear a little click of the bar pushing up into the loaded plates. This is referred to as taking the slack out of the bar.

2. Maintaining the stiff and neutral to slightly arched (not rounded) back position, push into the floor with your feet, allowing your hips, shoulders, and the bar to all rise at the same rate until the bar passes the knees.

3. The bar should travel as close to your legs as possible without adding extra resistance.

4. Once the bar passes your knees proceed to extend your hips until you are completely erect *(b)*.

5. Return to the floor by following the exact same path as you lower the bar to the floor.

VARIATION EXECUTION

Your range of motion while maintaining a neutral spine might prevent you from returning to the floor when performing the deadlift with two dumbbells or kettlebells or a single dumbbell *(d)*. Try to achieve the same depth as you would with the barbell and bumper plates.

COMMON FAULTS

- *Rounding of the back.*
    - Focus on tightening your lats.
    - Try to maintain whole-foot pressure (maybe even favoring the heels a bit more).
    - Take the slack out of the bar, or create and maintain total-body tension.
- *Trying to jerk the bar off the floor in the beginning of the lift.* Reexamine your efforts at creating and maintaining full-body pressure and pushing the floor away.
- *Hips rising sooner than the bar and shoulders.* Focus on full-body tension and on pushing the floor away as opposed to picking the bar up.
- *Not initiating the lowering of the bar by pushing the hips backward.* This is as simple as remembering to think about it. It is important for maintaining safe positions in the descent.

SUMO DEADLIFT

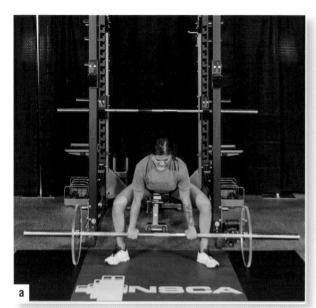
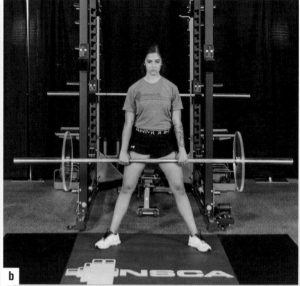

SETUP

1. Stand with your feet further than shoulder-width apart.

2. Feet are typically turned out to a 15- to 30-degree angle.

3. The bar is aligned over the feet and right next to, if not touching, your shins.

4. Your arms are in between your legs, with the grip aligned on the edge of the bar's knurling and not closer. (Knurling assists with grip.) Generally, your hands should be directly under your shoulders.

5. Using the bar to leverage yourself down, and pushing your knees outward, get into the bottom (beginning) position *(a)*.

   □ Knees should be aligned over your ankles or heels.

   □ Shins should be vertical (perpendicular to the floor).

   □ Shoulders should be over the bar.

   □ The hip position is dependent on your build, but they are generally higher than your knees and below your shoulders.

   □ Maintain a neutral to slightly arched (not rounded) spine.

   □ Keep your feet flat on the floor.

VARIATION SETUP

1. Kettlebells, dumbbells, and sandbags will require grip width adjustment and possibly a deeper bottom position because their handles are lower to the floor. The bottom position should not compromise the integrity of a neutral spine, so raise the "floor" as needed to be able to safely use these pieces of equipment.

2. If using a band, it will loop under the feet with the remainder of the setup unchanged. Adjust where you grip the band to determine the amount of resistance, keeping in mind it will be greatest at the top or lockout position.

EXECUTION

1. Take the slack out of the bar by tightening the lats and putting pressure into the floor with your feet. To take the slack out of the bar, use the bar to lower yourself down into the beginning position, creating full-body tension. You should hear a little click of the bar pushing up into the loaded plates. This is referred to as taking the slack out of the bar.

2. Maintaining the neutral to slightly arched (not rounded) back position, push into the floor with your feet, allowing your hips, shoulders, and the bar to all rise at the same rate until the bar passes the knees.

3. The bar should travel as close to your legs as possible without adding extra resistance.

4. Once the bar passes your knees proceed to extend your hips until you are completely erect *(b)*.

5. Return to the floor by following the exact same path as you lower the bar to the floor.

VARIATION EXECUTION

Your range of motion while maintaining a neutral spine might prevent you from returning to the floor when performing the deadlift with two dumbbells or kettlebells. Try to achieve the same depth as you would with the barbell and bumper plates.

COMMON FAULTS

■ *Rounding of the back.*
  □ Focus on tightening your lats.
  □ Try to maintain whole-foot pressure (maybe even favoring the heels a bit more).
  □ Take the slack out of the bar, or create and maintain total-body tension.

■ *Trying to jerk the bar off the floor in the beginning of the lift.* Reexamine your efforts at creating and maintaining full-body pressure and pushing the floor away.

■ *Hips rising sooner than the bar and shoulders.* Focus on full-body tension and on pushing the floor away as opposed to picking the bar up.

■ *Not initiating the lowering of the bar by pushing the hips backward.* This is as simple as remembering to think about it. It is important for maintaining safe positions in the descent.

■ *Starting with hips too low or treating the beginning position like the bottom position of a squat.* Make sure your hips are above your knees in the beginning position.

TRAP BAR DEADLIFT

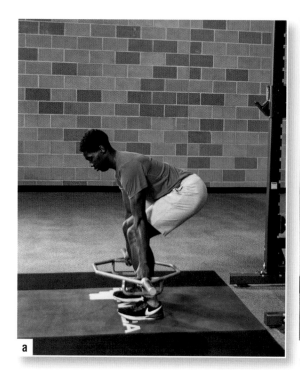
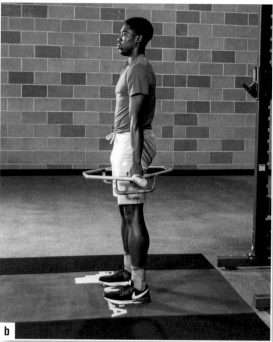

While this exercise is very similar to the deadlift, it is described in detail separately because it is also an event on the ACFT.

SETUP

1. Step near the center of the bar.

2. Align yourself so that your mid-foot (or where your shoelaces are tied) is in line with the center of the bar sleeves.

3. The feet are hip- to shoulder-width apart.

4. The feet can be straight ahead or turned out to a 15-degree angle.

5. Grab the handles and align your grip so that your hands are in line with the center of the bar sleeves. (Surprisingly, this is often overlooked.)

6. Use the bar to lower yourself down into the beginning position, creating full-body tension. You should hear a little click of the bar pushing up into the loaded plates. This is referred to as taking the slack out of the bar.

7. The hip position is dependent on your build, but your hips are generally higher than your knees and below your shoulders.

8. Maintain a neutral to slightly arched (not rounded) spine.

9. Keep your feet flat on the floor with whole-foot pressure.

EXECUTION

1. Take the slack out of the bar by tightening the lats and putting pressure into the floor with your feet *(a)*. (These notes were mentioned in the setup but are often forgotten once execution begins; they are so beneficial that we mention them twice.)

2. Maintaining the neutral to slightly arched (not rounded) back position, drive your feet into the floor, allowing your hips, shoulders, and the bar to all rise at the same rate. Think of pushing the floor away.

3. The bar should travel in a straight line until the hips and knees are fully extended and you are completely erect *(b)*.

4. Return the bar to the floor by following the exact same path in the descent, starting by pushing your hips backward slightly.

COMMON FAULTS

- *Rounding of the back.*
   - Focus on tightening your lats.
   - Try to maintain whole-foot pressure (maybe even favoring the heels a bit more).
   - Take the slack out of the bar, or create and maintain total-body tension.

- *Trying to jerk the bar off the floor in the beginning of the lift.* Reexamine your efforts at creating and maintaining full-body pressure and pushing the floor away.

- *Hips rising sooner than the bar and shoulders.* Focus on full-body tension and on pushing the floor away as opposed to picking the bar up.

- *Not initiating the lowering of the bar by pushing hips backward.* This is as simple as remembering to think about it. It is important for maintaining safe positions in the descent.

ROMANIAN DEADLIFT

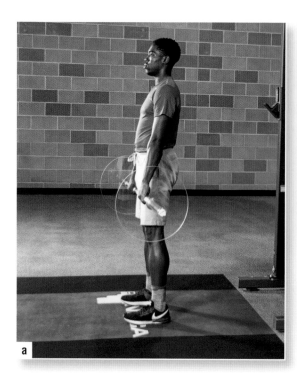
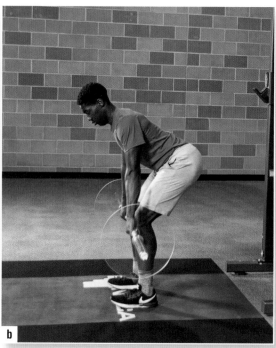

SETUP

1. Grip a barbell at a width just outside your hips, typically about a thumb's length from the smooth center of the bar.

2. Feet are hip- to shoulder-width apart and in a neutral position or just slightly turned outward.

3. Slightly bend the knees.

4. Maintain a neutral to slightly arched (not rounded) spine.

5. Keep your feet flat on the floor with whole-foot pressure.

VARIATION SETUP

1. Your stance remains the same regardless of variation, but kettlebells, dumbbells, or band handles will be held at your side to keep them as close to your center of mass as possible.

2. If using a band, loop it under your feet and adjust your grip to increase or decrease the resistance, keeping in mind that the resistance is greatest at the top or lockout positions.

EXECUTION

1. Tighten your lats by squeezing your upper arms toward your torso as though trying to seal your armpits shut *(a)*.

2. Maintain a neutral to slightly arched (not rounded) spine as you push your hips backward, allowing the hips to flex.

3. As the hips flex the barbell should slide down the front of your legs.

4. The slight knee bend created in the setup should remain constant, allowing most of the movement to happen at the hips.

5. The weight should shift toward your heels, but make sure you maintain whole-foot pressure, including keeping the big toes on the ground.

6. Continue to allow the barbell to travel down your legs, while maintaining proper back alignment, until you feel a stretch in your hamstrings or the backs of your legs *(b)*.

7. Once you feel the stretch, reverse the action by pushing or driving your feet into the floor and extending your hips until fully erect.

COMMON FAULTS

- *Rounding of the back.*
  - □ Focus on tightening your lats.
  - □ Try to maintain whole-foot pressure (maybe even favoring the heels a bit more).
  - □ Reexamine your thoughts around initiating the movement. Push the hips backward as opposed to thinking about simply bending forward . . . or not thinking at all.
- *Going too low.* This is indicated by a rounding of your lower back. Remember to stop the descent when you feel a stretch. Any extra range of motion past that stretch is most likely coming from spinal flexion.
- *Bending the knees too much.* Push your hips back as opposed to squatting down. Do not allow the knees to bend so that you can use more weight or so the exercise feels less difficult.
- *Barbell traveling away from your legs.* Initiate the movement by pushing your hips backward.

SINGLE-LEG ROMANIAN DEADLIFT

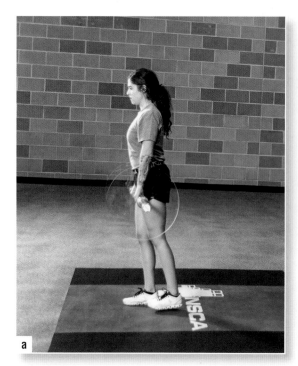
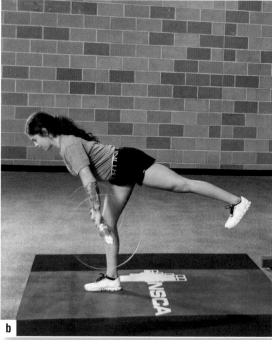

SETUP

1. Grip a barbell at a width just outside your hips, typically about a thumb's length from the smooth center of the bar.

2. Feet are hip- to shoulder-width apart and in a neutral position or just slightly turned outward.

3. Slightly bend the knees.

4. Maintain a neutral to slightly arched (not rounded) spine.

5. Keep your feet flat on the floor with whole-foot pressure.

VARIATION SETUP

1. Your stance remains the same regardless of variation, but kettlebells, dumbbells, or band handles will be held at your side to keep them as close to your center of mass as possible.

2. If using a band, loop it under your stance foot and adjust your grip to increase or decrease the resistance, keeping in mind that the resistance is greatest at the top or lockout positions.

3. When holding the resistance in only one hand, use the hand on the same side as the leg that is not in contact with the floor.

EXECUTION

1. Maintain a neutral to slightly arched (not rounded) spine as you push your hips backward, allowing the hip of the down leg to flex as the opposite leg stays in line with the torso *(a)*.

2. As the hip of the down leg flexes, the barbell should travel down your legs with your arms fully extended.

3. The slight knee bend created in the setup should remain constant in the down leg, allowing most of the movement to happen at the hip.

4. The weight should shift toward your heels, but make sure you maintain whole-foot pressure, including keeping the big toes on the floor.

5. Continue to allow the barbell to travel downward, while maintaining proper back alignment and position of the rear leg, until you feel a stretch in your hamstrings or the backs of your down leg *(b)*.

6. Once you feel the stretch, reverse the action by pushing or driving your foot into the floor and extending your hips until you are fully erect, besides the slight knee bend that should be maintained throughout.

7. Perform all programmed repetitions on one side before performing them on the opposite side.

VARIATION EXECUTION

Using resistance in one arm should not change your position throughout the movement, so fight the natural tendency to rotate away from the side that is loaded.

COMMON FAULTS

- *Rounding of the back.*
  - Try to maintain whole-foot pressure (maybe even favoring the heels a bit more).
  - Reexamine your thoughts around initiating the movement. Push the hips backward as opposed to thinking about simply bending forward . . . or not thinking at all.
- *Going too low.* This is indicated by a rounding of your lower back. Remember to stop the descent when you feel a stretch. Any extra range of motion past that stretch is most likely coming from spinal flexion.
- *Bending the knee too much.* Push your hips back as opposed to squatting down. Do not allow the knee to bend so that you can use more weight or so the exercise feels less difficult.

STABILITY BALL LEG CURL

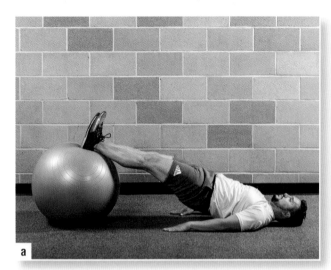
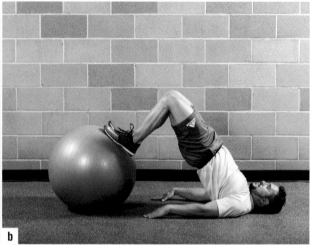

SETUP

1. Lay down with your back to the floor.

2. Position the stability ball so that your heels and lower calves are on top of the ball.

3. Rest your arms on the floor between a 45- and 90-degree angle from your torso.

4. Extend your hips by driving your heels and lower calves into the ball. Now your ankles, knees, hips, and shoulders should all be in a straight line *(a)*.

VARIATION SETUP

1. Heels can be placed in suspension trainer loops 12 inches (30 cm) off the floor, on sliders, or even on towels on a smooth surface such as a gym floor *(c-d)*.

2. If using a single leg, keep the hips level while the nonworking leg is kept straight and suspended in the air.

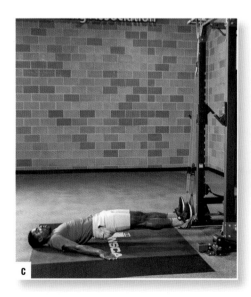
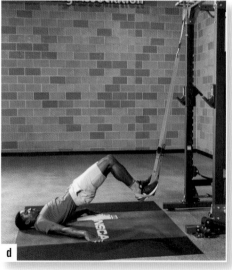

EXECUTION

1. Drive your heels and lower calves into the stability ball, allowing your knees to flex so the ball rolls toward your torso.

2. Continue on this path until your shins are almost perpendicular to the floor or you cannot roll any further.

3. As your knees flex and the stability ball rolls toward your torso, your body should elevate, with your knees, hips, and shoulders aligned *(b)*.

VARIATION EXECUTION

Mirror movements from the stability ball execution when using the suspension trainer for the variation exercise.

COMMON FAULT

- *Starting the movement by flexing the hips.*
  - ☐ Focus on driving your heels into the stability ball to elevate your body rather than simply curling the ball toward you.
  - ☐ Keep the hips engaged so they do not flex.

GLUTE-HAM RAISE

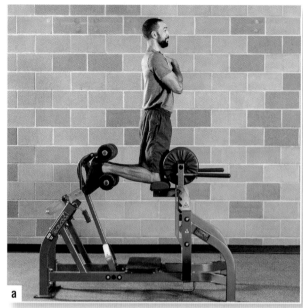

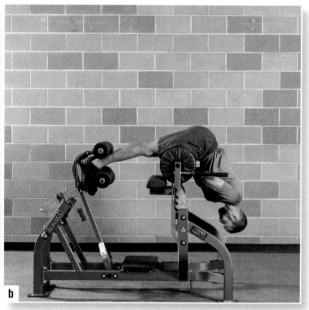

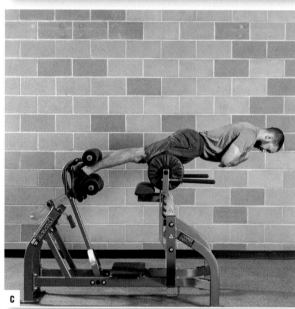

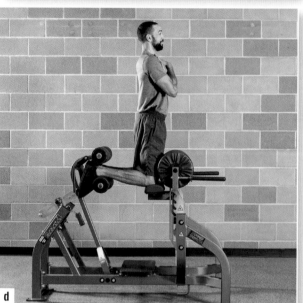

SETUP

1. Set up the glute-ham raise bench so that your feet are as far away from the pad as possible while your knees are still in contact with it so that you do not slide down.

2. Start in the upright position, where your thighs and torso are in alignment and perpendicular to the floor *(a)*.

3. If adding weight, hold it close to your torso.

EXECUTION

1. Keeping your hips engaged so that your thighs and torso stay in a straight line, allow your body to move forward and then downward, pushing yourself away from the bench and allowing the knees to extend.

2. Once your torso is parallel to the floor and your knees can no longer extend, allow your hips to flex until your torso is upside down and perpendicular to the floor *(b)*.

3. Once you have reached this bottom position, reverse the action in a similar smoothly segmented fashion. First extend the hips until the body is parallel to the floor *(c)*. Then flex the knees to bring the body back to the initial upright position, keeping the torso and thighs in line with each other *(d)*.

COMMON FAULTS

- *Starting the movement by flexing the hips.* Reexamine the intent to push your hips into the pad as if pushing yourself away from the machine.

- *Initiating the return to the beginning position by flexing your knees first.*
    - Wait to flex the knees until the body is parallel to the floor.
    - If you cannot return to the starting position without bending your knees first, the exercise might be too difficult. You can perform each repetition in an eccentric (downward motion)–only fashion until you build the strength, or you could substitute the stability ball leg curl exercise.

HIP BRIDGE

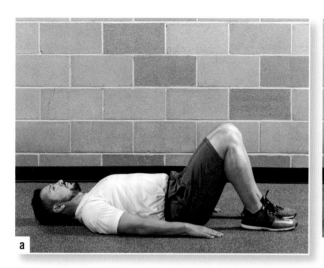
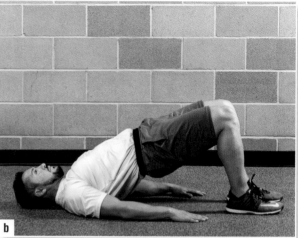

SETUP

1. Lay on your back and bend your knees to 90 degrees with your feet flat on the floor.

2. Keep your feet about 12 inches (30 cm) apart so they are slightly outside of your knees and your knees are slightly wider than your hips.

3. Your head should be relaxed on the floor, and your arms should be out to your side at 45 degrees or less *(a)*.

VARIATION SETUP

1. If your feet are in a suspension trainer, the loops should be about 12 inches (30 cm) off the floor.

2. To increase the difficulty, you can place the feet on top of a stability ball; add a load across the front of your hips using a barbell *(c)*, kettlebell, or dumbbell; use one leg instead of two; or place your upper back on a bench.

3. If using a band as resistance, hold each end of the band at your side with the band resting across the front of your hips.

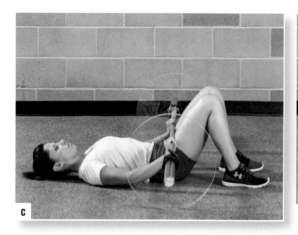
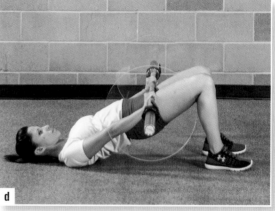

EXECUTION

1. Drive your heels down and your hips up until you are locked out in a bridge position *(b)*.
2. Squeeze your butt in the top position and keep your abdominals tight to avoid arching your lower back excessively.
3. Keep a fairly straight line from each foot to your hip.
4. Lower down under control as if your hips were a hinge closing.

VARIATION EXECUTION

If your feet are on a stability ball or suspension trainer, do not let them move away from your butt. When executing the variation, your knees should stay fixed at 90 degrees *(d)*.

COMMON FAULTS

- *Excessively arching your back.* Initiate movement through your hips and keep your abdominals tight throughout the movement. You should not be able to see your ribs flair.
- *Letting the knees flail outward.* Maintain a straight line from your feet through your hips, and lightly squeeze a medicine ball or something of a similar size between your legs.

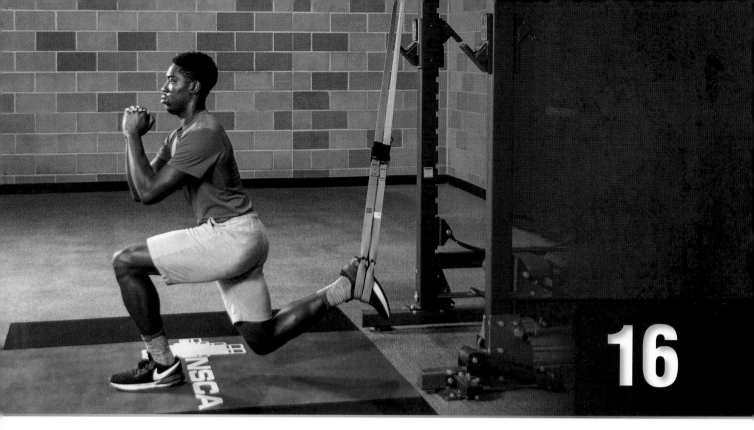

16

Lower Body Pushing Exercises

Squats and lunges build leg strength and muscular endurance, depending on the volume and intensity prescribed. They transfer directly to the MDL, SPT, and SDC but also strongly support the 2MR. In the absence of a barbell and squat stand or rack, single-leg and lunge variations can provide a decent substitute to the back squat exercise as well as deadlift exercises. While these exercises mostly use dumbbells and barbells, kettlebells and other weighted pieces of equipment can easily be substituted in the absence of more traditional training equipment.

Lower Body Pushing Exercises Finder

ALTERNATIVE LOWER BODY PUSHING EXERCISES

The lower body pushing exercises included in the chapter 12 programs are the most preferred exercises as they relate to the ACFT. If you do not have the needed equipment to do a preferred exercise, you will need to choose an alternative exercise. Go to table 16.1 and find the exercise you need to replace along the top row. (The name will not include the piece of equipment.) Next, find the equipment options to which you have access along the left column. Your alternative exercise options are where the column of the exercise you are replacing intersects the rows of the types of equipment you have access to. Choose the option that best mimics the position, movement, and resistance level of the preferred exercise in the chapter 12 programs. Note that not every type of equipment supports an alternative exercise, but at least one bodyweight replacement exists for every exercise, so there is no excuse to entirely omit a programmed exercise.

Table 16.1 Alternative Lower Body Pushing Exercises

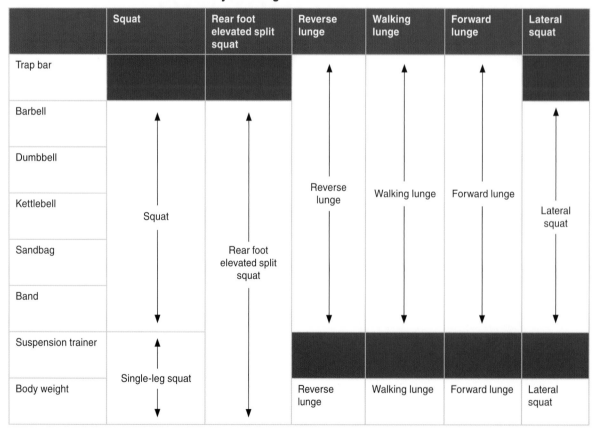

METHODS OF ADDING LOAD OR RESISTANCE FOR LOWER BODY PUSHING EXERCISES

Figures 16.1*a* through 16.1*k* show a variety of ways to load or add resistance to lower body pushing exercises based on what piece of equipment is available to you. Many of the lower body pushing exercises can use several, if not all, of the loading options. Choose the load and position that best maximizes the resistance for the number of repetitions assigned within the program.

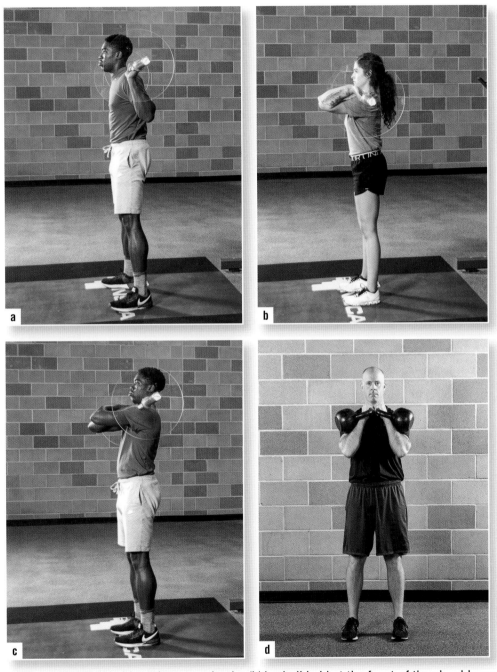

Figure 16.1 *(a)* Barbell held on the upper back, *(b)* barbell held at the front of the shoulders with a parallel-arm grip, *(c)* barbell held at the front of the shoulders with a crossed-arm grip, *(d)* kettle-bells held at the front of the shoulders (front racked),

(continued)

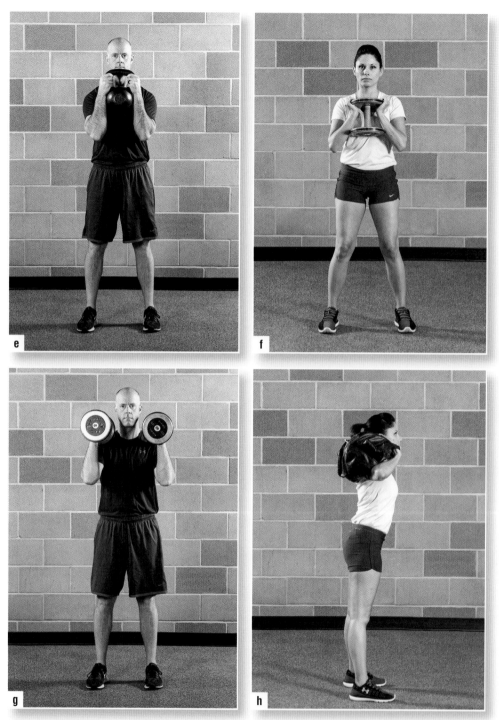

Figure 16.1 *(continued)*   *(e)* kettlebell held in a goblet position, *(f)* dumbbell held in a goblet position, *(g)* dumbbells held at the shoulders, *(h)* sandbag held on the back,

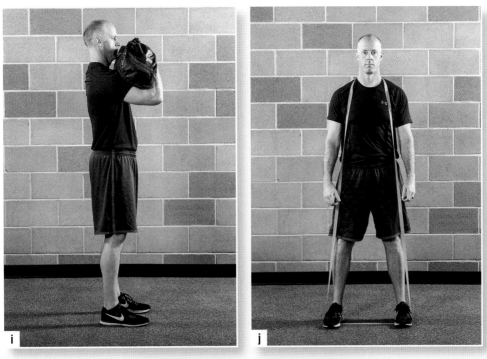

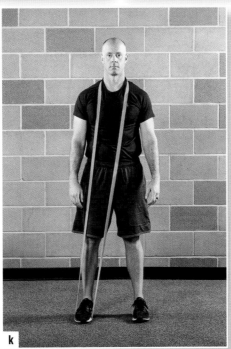

Figure 16.1 *(continued)* *(i)* sandbag held in the front, *(j)* band in a squat setup, *(k)* setup of a band for a single-leg squat or lunge (all versions).

SQUAT

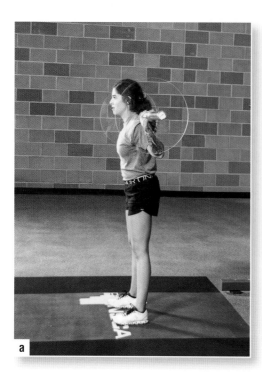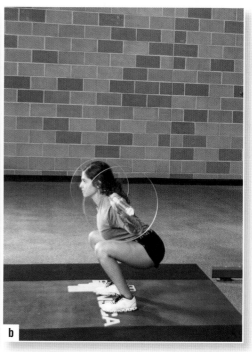

SETUP

1. Make sure the bar is set up in the rack (not seen in the photos, but still needed) so that you must lower your body only slightly to step under the bar. The bar height in the rack should not be at a height that forces you to go up on your toes to get the bar off the hooks.

2. Facing the bar and the rack, grab the bar with a grip width outside your shoulders but as close as possible based on your specific mobility and comfort level.

3. Step under the bar, making sure your body is centered on the bar.

4. The bar should be placed on the shoulders or back in the natural groove created between the traps and the rear deltoid. (Optimal placement of the bar can depend on the intent of the exercise and the individual, but the most common style is referred to as the *athletic squat.*)

5. Make sure that both feet are under the bar before lifting the bar off the hooks.

6. Create tension or brace to prepare to lift the bar off the hooks, then lift the bar off the hooks and take as few steps backward as possible to get in position to squat without hitting the hooks on the way up or down. (To clearly show the movement, the exercise was photographed outside of the squat rack.)

7. The feet should be aligned at shoulder width or slightly wider.

8. The feet should be angled anywhere from neutral (straight ahead) to turned out at a 30-degree angle.

9. Maintain a neutral to slightly arched (not rounded) spine position.

10. Keep the feet flat on the floor with whole-foot pressure.

VARIATION SETUP

1. A single kettlebell can be held in a goblet position, or two kettlebells can be held in the front rack position or at your sides with your elbows straight.

2. A single dumbbell can be held in a goblet position, or two dumbbells can be held vertically on your shoulders or in the front.

3. A barbell can be front loaded instead of back loaded.

4. A sandbag can be front loaded or back loaded.

5. A band can be routed under the middle of each foot, over the shoulders, and behind the neck.

EXECUTION

1. Brace or create tension in the torso in preparation to support the weight. Maintain a neutral or slightly rounded (not arched) spine position *(a)*.

2. Simultaneously flex the knees and hips as you descend downward, and push back slightly with your hips.

3. The knees track in line with your feet; do not let them cave inward.

4. The feet remain flat on the floor with whole-foot pressure.

5. Go as low as you can while maintaining the integrity of the neutral spine, as well as proper ankle, knee, and hip alignment *(b)*.

6. Return to the beginning position by pushing or driving your feet into the floor to push your body away or upward until hips and knees are fully extended.

VARIATION EXECUTION

Variations should not greatly alter execution with the exception of the selected piece of equipment remaining in the same position on or near the body as it starts. For example, the elbows should remain high with the barbell securely supported by the shoulders when front loaded.

COMMON FAULTS

■ *Not going low enough.* Have someone watch you from the side to make sure you are at least going low enough to have your hips in line, which should be parallel to the floor.
  □ If you cannot at least go that low while maintaining a neutral spine, be more conscious of the effort to drive your knees out throughout the entire movement.
  □ If that heightened consciousness does not fix the issue, you should only go as low as you can while maintaining a neutral spine position.

■ *Going lower than proper alignment allows.*
  □ Ensure that your upper or lower back does not begin to round, or that your ankles, knees, and hips do not lose proper alignment.
  □ Simply stop the descent sooner to prevent this from happening.

■ *Heels coming off the floor.*
  □ Try to sit backward slightly on your descent.
  □ Maintain whole-foot pressure on the descent and ascent, and to help correct the issue, consider focusing on more pressure through the heels throughout the movement.

■ *Hips rising too soon in ascent.*
  □ Reexamine your intent to push the entire body away from the floor on the ascent.
  □ Focus on keeping your chest up during the ascent.

SINGLE-LEG SQUAT

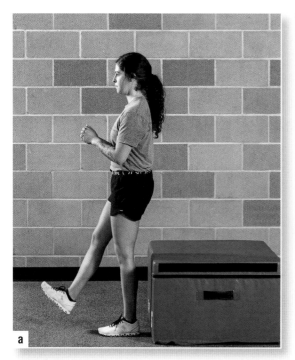
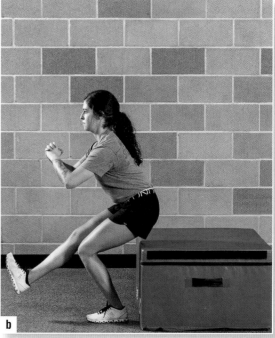

SETUP

1. Select a box or bench that allows you to sit on it with the midline of your thigh parallel to the floor.
2. Stand roughly one to two shoe lengths from the box or bench with your back facing it. The distance from the box or bench may need to be adjusted, but this is a good starting point.
3. The feet should be hip-width apart and pointed forward.

VARIATION SETUP

1. In the absence of a box or bench, any solid object about knee height can be used as a substitute.
2. A suspension trainer or band can be used without a box by holding the handles at chest height *(c)*.

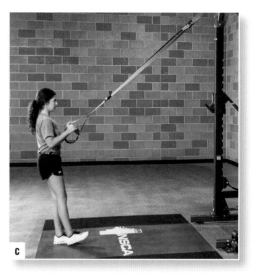

EXECUTION

1. Raise one foot off the ground, with that leg straight and moving forward slightly *(a)*.

2. The foot remaining on the ground should maintain whole-foot pressure, pressing into the ground.

3. With your arms extended out in front of you to assist with balance, allow the hip and knee of the down leg to flex as you lower into the single-leg squat *(b)*.

4. Control the descent to prevent falling or collapsing to the box or bench, and barely touch the top surface before reversing the action.

5. Once you touch the box or bench, drive your foot into the floor with whole-foot pressure and think about pushing the floor away.

6. Continue driving your foot into the floor until the hip and knee are fully extended.

VARIATION EXECUTION

If holding a suspension trainer or band for assistance, let the arms straighten as you descend *(d)* and use only as much assistance as needed to complete the movement when pulling with the arms to help on the way back up.

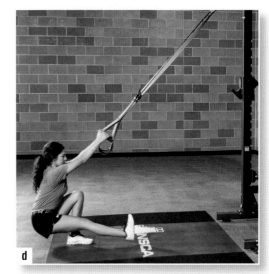

COMMON FAULTS

- *Heel coming off the ground.*
  - □ Focus on maintaining whole-foot pressure and driving into the ground throughout the entire movement.
  - □ Sit or shift your weight backward more in the initial decent into the single-leg squat, and maintain that shift throughout the movement.

- *Bouncing off the box or bench.* Reexamine your effort to barely touch the top surface. The action of deceleration and reversing the action is a desired muscle action, and you want to avoid assistance by bouncing off the box or bench.

REAR FOOT ELEVATED SPLIT SQUAT

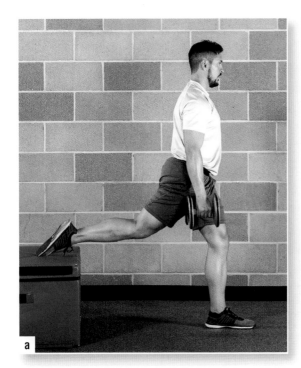
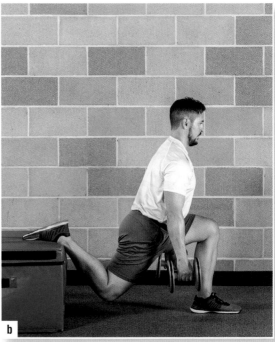

SETUP

1. Set up a box, bench, or box (from here on referred to as a *box*) that is mid-shin to just below knee height.

2. Place the top of the foot, where the shoelaces would be or are, on the box.

3. Adjust the front foot so that it is 2 to 3 feet (0.6-0.9 m) in front of the box.

4. Keeping your rear foot on the box, perform a single squat until the back knee touches the floor.

5. Adjust your front foot so that you feel comfortable and so that your knee is somewhere between directly over your ankle to right behind your toes *(a)*.

6. Make note of this foot position for all subsequent sets.

7. Return to the beginning position.

VARIATION SETUP

1. A single kettlebell can be held in a goblet position, or two kettlebells can be held in the front rack position or at your sides with your arms extended.

2. A single dumbbell can be held in a goblet position, or two dumbbells can be held vertically on your shoulders.

3. A barbell can be front loaded instead of back loaded.

4. A sandbag can be front loaded or back loaded.

5. A band can be routed under the middle of the lead foot and over the shoulders but behind the neck.

6. The rear foot can be elevated in a suspension trainer loop *(c)*.

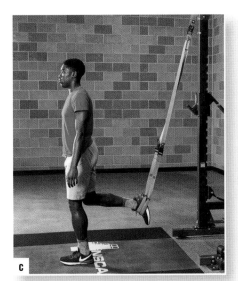
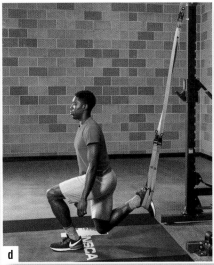

EXECUTION

1. Start the movement by allowing the front leg's knee and hip to flex as you descend into a single-leg squat position, maintaining whole-foot pressure into the floor.

2. Proceed with this action until the back knee barely touches the floor (good physical indicator of proper depth).

3. The knee of the front leg should track over the foot and remain somewhere between the ankle and the toes of that foot *(b)*.

4. Once the back knee barely touches the ground, drive the front foot into the floor with whole-foot pressure, reversing the action.

5. Continue to drive into the floor until the hip and knee are fully extended and you are back to the beginning position.

VARIATION EXECUTION

Variations should not greatly alter execution with the exception of the selected piece of equipment remaining in the same position as it starts. For example, the elbows should remain high with the barbell securely supported by the shoulders when front loaded, or your rear foot should remain in the same position in a suspension trainer *(d)*.

COMMON FAULTS

■ *Maintaining incorrect positioning.* Most faults are associated with the positioning. Understand that you are not locked into your initial foot position; you can adjust for proper setup and distance from the anchor point.

■ *Bouncing the knee off the floor.* Reexamine your effort to barely touch the back knee to the floor. Not only is the action of deceleration and reversing the action desirable, but this will help prevent injury to the knee.

REVERSE LUNGE

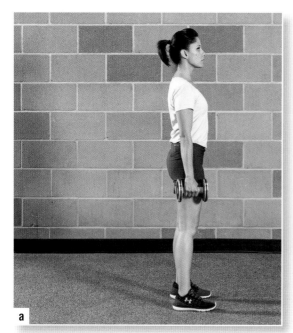
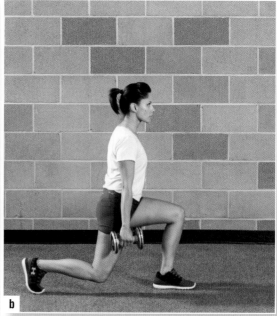

SETUP

Stand with your feet hip- to shoulder-width apart *(a)*.

VARIATION SETUP

1. A single kettlebell can be held in a goblet position, or two kettlebells can be held in the front rack position or at your sides with your arms long.

2. A single dumbbell can be held in a goblet position, or two dumbbells can be held vertically on your shoulders.

3. A barbell can be front loaded instead of back loaded.

4. A sandbag can be front loaded or back loaded.

5. A band can be routed under the middle of the lead foot and over the shoulders but behind the neck.

EXECUTION

1. Brace or create tension in the torso in preparation to support the weight. Maintain a neutral or slightly arched (not rounded) spine position.

2. Lunge backward with one foot, allowing the front leg to support your weight as the movement occurs.

3. Simultaneously, as you lunge backward, the front leg's hip, knee, and ankle flex, allowing your center of gravity to move closer to the ground.

4. As the rear foot contacts the ground, the front leg's knee should be flexed to nearly 90 degrees.

5. Descending in a controlled manner, stop once the rear leg's knee barely touches the ground *(b)*.

6. Once the back knee barely touches the ground, drive your front foot into the ground with whole-foot pressure, pushing the entire body up and back to the beginning position, bringing your back leg underneath you.

VARIATION EXECUTION

Variations should not greatly alter execution with the exception of the selected piece of equipment remaining in the same position as it starts. For example, the elbows should remain high with the barbell securely supported by the shoulders when front loaded.

COMMON FAULTS

- *Bouncing the knee off the ground.* Reexamine your effort to barely touch the back knee to the floor. Not only is the action of deceleration and reversing the action desirable, but this will help prevent injury to the knee.

- *Stepping too far back.* Pay attention to the position of the knee as it relates to your ankle. If it is even slightly behind center, it is too far, and you should reduce the length of your step.

- *Not stepping back far enough.* Pay attention to the position of the knee as it relates to your toes. If it is ahead of your toes or if your heel comes off the ground, take a longer step back.

- *Segmenting the movement.*
    - On the lunging action, focus on flexing the knee and hip simultaneously as opposed to stepping back then down.
    - On the returning action, focus on pushing the body up as you simultaneously bring your back leg underneath your hips.

WALKING LUNGE

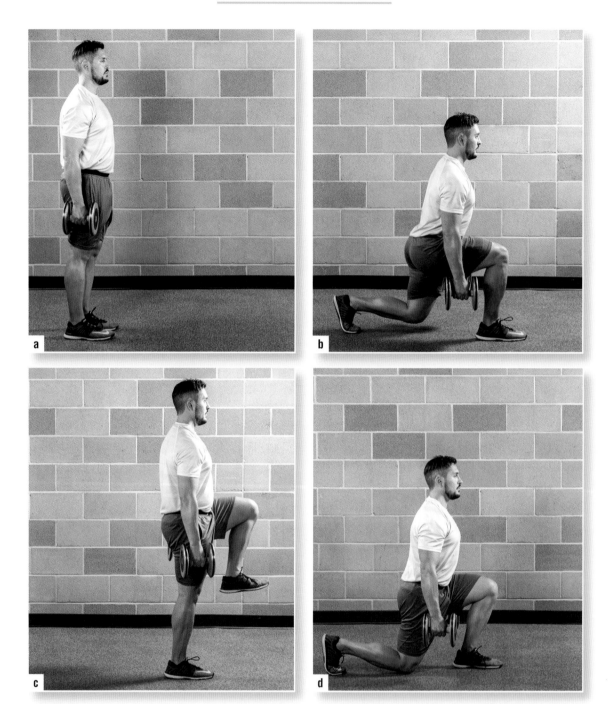

SETUP

Stand with your feet hip- to shoulder-width apart *(a)*.

VARIATION SETUP

1. A single kettlebell can be held in a goblet position, or two kettlebells can be held in the front rack position or at your sides with your arms long.
2. A single dumbbell can be held in a goblet position, or two dumbbells can be held vertically on your shoulders.
3. A barbell can be front loaded instead of back loaded.
4. A sandbag can be front loaded or back loaded.
5. A band can be routed under the middle of the lead foot and over the shoulders but behind the neck.

EXECUTION

1. Brace or create tension in the torso in preparation to support the weight. Maintain a neutral or slightly arched (not rounded) spine position.
2. Lunge forward with what becomes your front foot, anticipating the flexion of both the knee and hip upon the foot's contact with the floor.
3. As the foot contacts the floor, both the knee and hip should flex simultaneously to absorb the force.
4. Allow this to take place until the thigh's midline is parallel to the floor or until the knee of the back leg barely touches the floor *(b)*.
5. Once the back knee barely touches the floor, drive into the floor with whole-foot pressure, pushing the entire body upward as the back leg travels underneath the hips *(c)*.
6. Once you are back to the initial beginning position, go back to step 1 with the other leg *(d)*.

VARIATION EXECUTION

Variations should not greatly alter execution with the exception of the selected piece of equipment remaining in the same position as it starts. For example, the elbows should remain high with the barbell securely supported by the shoulders when front loaded.

COMMON FAULTS

■ *Bouncing the knee off the floor.* Reexamine your effort to barely touch the back knee to the floor. Not only is the action of deceleration and reversing the action desirable, but this will help prevent injury to the knee.

■ *Stepping too far forward.*
   □ Pay attention to the position of the knee as it relates to your ankle. If it is even slightly behind center, it is too far, and you should reduce the length of your step.
   □ Examine the arch of your lower back. If the lower back arches as you lunge into position, you are likely compensating for the need for hip extension. Reduce the length of your step so that your back leg's knee is close to or directly under your hips.

■ *Not lunging forward far enough.* Pay attention to the position of the knee as it relates to your toes. If your knee is ahead of your toes or if your heel comes off the floor, reduce the length of your step.

■ *Segmenting the movement.*
   □ On the lunging action focus on flexing the knee and hip simultaneously as opposed to stepping out then down.
   □ On the returning action, focus on pushing the body up and back simultaneously as opposed to up and then back.

FORWARD LUNGE

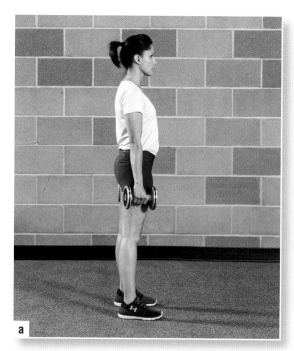
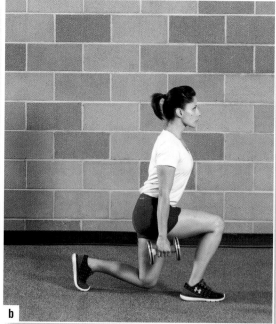

SETUP

Stand with your feet hip- to shoulder-width apart *(a)*.

VARIATION SETUP

1. A single kettlebell can be held in a goblet position, or two kettlebells can be held in the front rack position or at your sides with your arms long.

2. A single dumbbell can be held in a goblet position, or two dumbbells can be held vertically on your shoulders.

3. A barbell can be front loaded instead of back loaded.

4. A sandbag can be front loaded or back loaded.

5. A band can be routed under the middle of the lead foot and over the shoulders but behind the neck.

EXECUTION

1. Brace or create tension in the torso in preparation to support the weight. Maintain a neutral or slightly arched (not rounded) spine position.

2. Lunge forward with one foot, anticipating the flexion of both the knee and hip upon the foot's contact with the floor.

3. As the foot contacts the floor, both the knee and hip should flex simultaneously to absorb the force.

4. Allow this to take place until the thigh's midline is parallel to the floor or until the knee of the back leg barely touches the floor *(b)*.

5. Once the back knee barely touches the floor, drive your front foot into the floor with whole-foot pressure, pushing the entire body up and backward to the start position.

VARIATION EXECUTION

Variations should not greatly alter execution with the exception of the selected piece of equipment remaining in the same position as it starts. For example, the elbows should remain high with the barbell securely supported by the shoulders when front loaded.

COMMON FAULTS

- *Bouncing the knee off the floor.* Reexamine your effort to barely touch the back knee to the floor. Not only is the action of deceleration and reversing the action desirable, but this will help prevent injury to the knee.

- *Stepping too far forward.*
   - Pay attention to the position of the knee as it relates to your ankle. If it is even slightly behind center, it is too far, and you should reduce the length of your step.
   - Examine the arch of your lower back. If the lower back arches as you lunge into position, you are likely compensating for the need of hip extension. Reduce the length of your step so that your back leg's knee is close to or directly under your hips.

- *Not lunging forward far enough.* Pay attention to the position of the knee as it relates to your toes. If your knee is ahead of your toes or your heel comes off the floor, reduce the length of your step.

- *Segmenting the movement.*
   - On the lunging action focus on flexing the knee and hip simultaneously as opposed to stepping out then down.
   - On the returning action, focus on pushing the body up and back simultaneously as opposed to up and then back.

LATERAL SQUAT

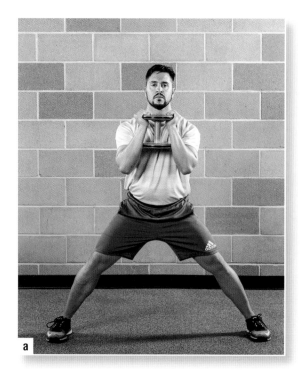 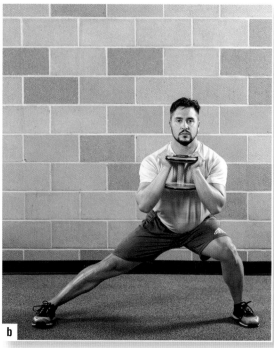

SETUP

1. Spread your legs so that each foot is 2 to 3 feet (0.6-0.9 m) wider than it would be in a normal standing position. This width will likely need to be adjusted to fit you and your body.

2. Start with your feet pointing straight ahead. They will likely need to be adjusted anywhere from this straight-ahead position *(a)* to a 30-degree outwardly (externally) rotated position depending on what best fits your body.

3. Proceed to sit down, back, and toward one leg, keeping the opposite leg straight, to a position where the midline of your thigh is parallel to the floor or lower and both heels are on the floor. In this bottom position make note of how it feels for you, and adjust the width of your stance and position of your feet to make it the most comfortable to you.

4. Perform step 3 for the other leg.

5. Make note of your foot position and width of your stance, and use this for your initial beginning position during execution.

VARIATION SETUP

1. A single kettlebell can be held in a goblet position, or two kettlebells can be held in the front rack position or at your sides with your arms long.

2. A single dumbbell can be held in a goblet position, or two dumbbells can be held vertically on your shoulders.

3. A barbell can be front loaded instead of back loaded.

4. A sandbag can be front loaded or back loaded.

5. A band can be routed under the middle of the lead foot and over the shoulders but behind the neck.

EXECUTION

1. Start the movement by sitting down, back, and toward one leg, keeping the opposite leg straight.

2. Continue the action of step 1 until the midline of the thigh that you are squatting toward is parallel to the floor or lower *(b)*.

3. Make sure that both heels stay in contact with the floor throughout the movement.

4. Once in the parallel or lower position, drive into the floor through your entire foot, pushing your body up and toward the beginning position.

5. Once back to the beginning position, execute all steps for the opposite leg.

VARIATION EXECUTION

Variations should not greatly alter execution with the exception of the selected piece of equipment remaining in the same position as it starts. For example, the elbows should remain high with the barbell securely supported by the shoulders when front loaded.

COMMON FAULTS

- *Not getting low enough.*
  - □ Reexamine the width needed to comfortably get to the parallel position.
  - □ Go lighter on the weight if needed.
- *Heels coming off the floor.*
  - □ Focus on the width needed to comfortably get to the parallel position; lack of range of motion in the hip can cause the heel to raise.
  - □ Focus on the foot placement needed to comfortably get to the parallel position; lack of ankle range of motion without an outwardly (externally) rotated foot can cause the heel to raise.

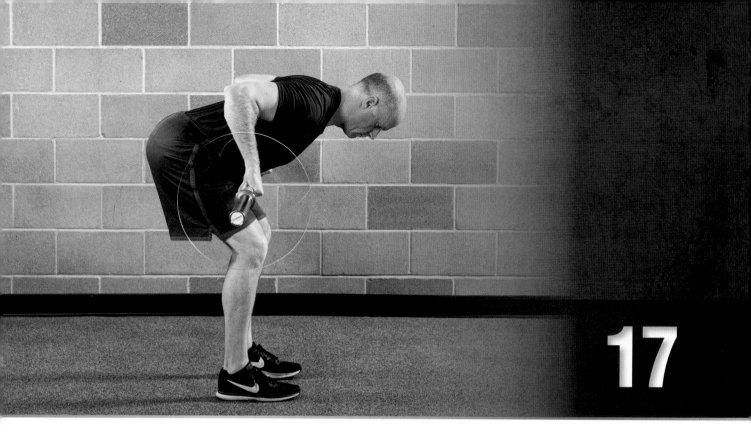

17

Upper Body Pulling Exercises

Upper body pulling exercises are used to increase back strength and muscular endurance. These exercises transfer directly to the LTK event but strongly support the physicality needed to be successful in the MDL and SDC while helping offset the high volume of upper body pushing exercises needed to pass the HRP event. While dumbbells and barbells are not always available, pulling exercises can easily be done with sandbags, kettlebells, suspension trainers, and bands.

Upper Body Pulling Exercises Finder

ALTERNATIVE UPPER BODY PULLING EXERCISES

The upper body pulling exercises included in the chapter 12 programs are the preferred exercises as they relate to the ACFT. If you do not have the needed equipment to do a preferred exercise, you will need to choose an alternative exercise. Go to table 17.1 and find the exercise you need to replace along the top row. (The name will not include the piece of equipment being used.) Next, find the equipment options to which you have access along the left-hand column. Your alternative exercise options are where the column of the exercise you are replacing intersects the rows of the types of equipment to which you have access. Choose the option that best mimics the position, movement, and resistance level of the preferred exercise in the chapter 12 programs. Note that not every type of equipment supports an alternative exercise, but at least one body weight replacement exists for every exercise, so there is no excuse to entirely omit a programmed exercise.

Table 17.1   Alternative Upper Body Pulling Exercises

	Chin-up	Pull-up	Bent-over row	Inverted row	Prone row	Biceps curl	Hammer curl	Band pull-apart	Rear delt raise	Facepull
Trap bar	↑	↑	↑	↑	↑					↑
Barbell						↑	Biceps curl			
Dumbbell	Bent-over row	Bent-over row			Prone row, bent-over row					Bent-over row
Kettlebell			Bent-over row	Bent-over row			Hammer curl	Rear delt raise	Rear delt raise	
Sandbag						Biceps curl				
Band	Pulldown	Pulldown	↓	↓	↓	↓	↓	Band pullapart	Band pullapart	↑
Suspension trainer	Inverted row	Inverted row	↑	↑	↑		Biceps curl	Rear delt raise	Rear delt raise	Facepull
Body weight	Chin-up*	Pull-up*	Inverted row ↓	Inverted row ↓	Inverted row ↓					Inverted row

*If these exercises cannot be performed with one's body weight due to a lack of strength, a band or partner can be used for assisted repetitions. (See the variation setup descriptions of each exercise for more detail.) A second option is to perform an eccentric-only version during which only the downward phase is performed. (Take three to five seconds to lower from a dead stop in the top position and maintain control throughout the descent.)

BAND PULLAPART

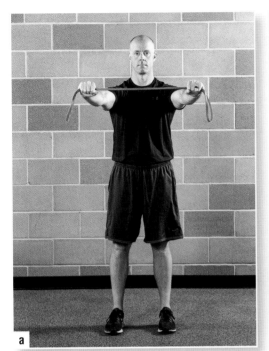
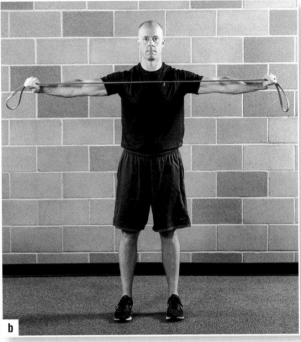

SETUP

1. Grasp a band so that your hands are shoulder-width apart in an overhand position. This grip width is a good beginning position; however, you may need to adjust your grip width based on strength and band tension. Also, you can use an underhand position on the band to do the reverse-grip pullapart.

2. Keeping your elbows extended, raise your arms in front of your torso until your wrists are level with your shoulders *(a)*.

3. The grip width should not be reduced from your initial beginning position. You always want to keep a little tension on the band, but do not let it go slack.

EXECUTION

1. Keeping your elbows fixed, pull the band apart by forcing your arms away from your midline *(b)*.

2. Once your elbows are in line with your shoulders, begin to follow the same path back toward your midline, controlling the return.

3. As your arms near your midline, remember to stop before the band becomes slack. You always want to keep tension on the band.

COMMON FAULTS

■ *Going too quickly.* Control the entire motion as the arms move away from your midline and as they return toward your midline.

■ *Raising your wrist above shoulder height.* Your arms should travel parallel to the floor. If you cannot maintain this position, you may need to reduce the band tension.

CHIN-UP

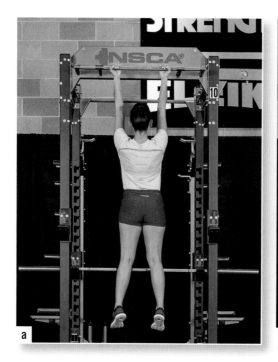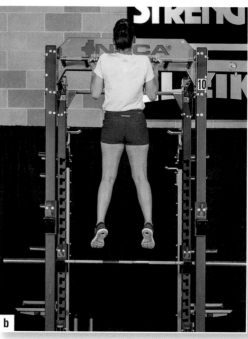

SETUP

1. Hold the bar underhand and with hands shoulder-width apart.

2. Hang from the bar with straight arms and with the feet off the floor. Keep the legs straight when possible *(a)*.

3. Maintain a neutral to slightly arched (not rounded) spine.

4. Keep your face forward with your chin parallel to the floor.

VARIATION SETUP

If this exercise cannot be performed with one's body weight due to a lack of strength, a band (girth hitched over the bar *[c]* or with a knee or feet in the band *[d]*) or partner can be used for assisted repetitions *(e)*. However, the band or partner should provide as little assistance as needed to complete the programmed repetitions.

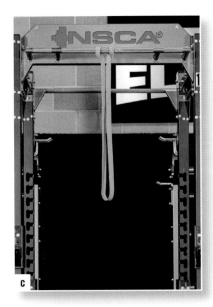
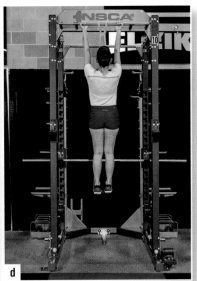
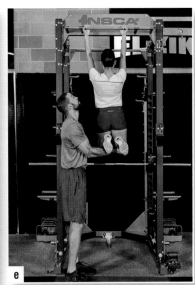

EXECUTION

1. Pull yourself up toward the bar, thinking about pulling the elbows down toward the floor and into your torso.

2. Pull yourself up until your chin clears the bar at a minimum, while keeping the chin parallel to the floor *(b)*.

3. Shoulder blades should drive down and slightly backward naturally. Finish at the top with a broad chest. Do not roll the shoulders forward.

4. Lower yourself following the same path until the arms are completely straight.

COMMON FAULTS

- *Trying to use momentum to facilitate the movement (kipping, kicking, swinging, etc.).* Focus on the controlled action of execution. If you still are unable to execute as described, reduce the weight. If you are using only body weight, reduce the weight by using a resistance band for assistance, an assisted pull-up machine, a partner supporting a portion of your weight, or a lat pulldown machine.

- *Not finishing with the chin over the bar.* Reduce the weight being used, as mentioned above.

- *Not straightening the arms completely at the bottom.* Be conscious of allowing them to extend, understanding the purpose is to train through the full range of motion.

- *Rolling shoulders forward.* Focus on the downward movement of the shoulders during the execution and allow them to travel slightly backward. This shrugging and rolling the shoulders forward can contribute to shoulder problems in the future.

PULL-UP

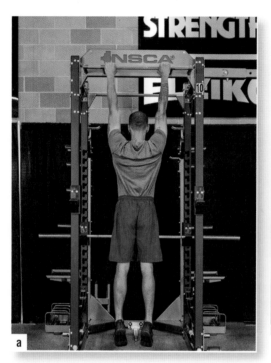
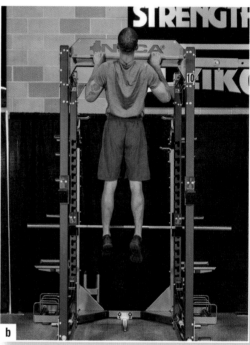

SETUP

1. Hold the bar overhand with hands slightly wider than shoulder width *(a)*.
2. Hang from the bar with straight arms and with feet off the floor. Keep the legs straight when possible.
3. Maintain a neutral to slightly arched (not rounded) spine.
4. Keep your face forward with your chin parallel to the floor.

VARIATION SETUP

1. To add weight, wear a pull-up belt with a chain attachment (and loop it through one or more weight plates or kettlebells), pinch a dumbbell handle between the feet, insert the foot or feet through the window of one or two kettlebells, or wear a weighted vest.
2. If this exercise cannot be performed with one's body weight due to a lack of strength, a band (girth hitched over the bar or with a knee or feet in the band) or partner can be used for assisted repetitions. (See photos in the chin-up exercise.) However, the band or partner should provide as little assistance as needed to complete the programmed repetitions.

EXECUTION

1. Pull yourself up toward the bar, thinking about pulling the elbows down toward the floor or your hips.

2. Keep your upper arms at about a 45-degree angle to your torso as you pull upward.

3. Pull yourself up until your chin clears the bar at a minimum. Keep the chin parallel to the floor *(b)*.

4. The shoulder blades should drive down and slightly backward naturally. Finish at the top with a broad chest. Do not roll the shoulders forward.

5. Lower yourself following the same path until the arms are completely straight.

COMMON FAULTS

- *Trying to use momentum to facilitate the movement (kipping, kicking, swinging, etc.).* Focus on the controlled action of execution. If you still are unable to execute as described, reduce the weight. If you are using only body weight, reduce the weight by using a resistance band for assistance, an assisted pull-up machine, a partner supporting a portion of your weight, or a lat pulldown machine.

- *Not finishing with the chin over the bar.* Reduce the weight being used, as mentioned above.

- *Not straightening the arms completely at the bottom.* Be conscious of allowing them to extend, understanding the purpose is to train through the full range of motion.

- *Rolling shoulders forward.* Focus on the downward movement of the shoulders during the execution and allow them to travel slightly backward. This shrugging and rolling the shoulders forward can contribute to shoulder problems in the future.

BENT-OVER ROW

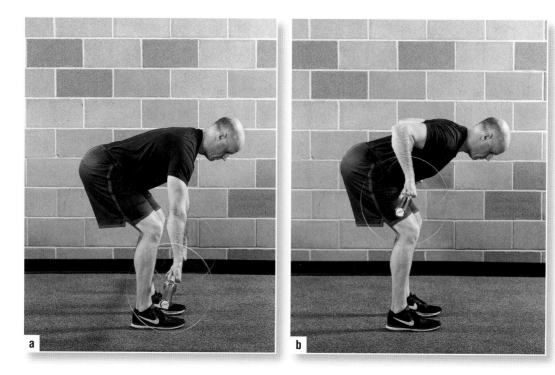

SETUP

1. Grab the bar with hands slightly wider than shoulder-width apart.

2. Get into a bent-over position by pushing your hips backward and allowing the knees to flex slightly.

3. Maintain a neutral to slightly arched (not rounded) spine.

4. Keep your head in a neutral position in line with your neutral spine.

5. Your back should be as close to parallel to the floor as possible while maintaining a neutral spine position *(a)*.

6. Your arms should be completely straight, with your hands in line with your shoulders.

VARIATION SETUP

1. Your grip might be normal (also called *overhand* or *pronated* as seen in the photos), reverse (also called *underhand* or *supinated*), or neutral (with the palms facing each other) when using different pieces of equipment to perform a bent-over row, such as a dumbbell.

2. The rest of the body position should remain the same as it is with the barbell version.

EXECUTION

1. Pull the bar up toward a place between the bottom of your chest and the bottom of your rib cage *(b)*.

2. The position of your back relative to the floor should remain constant throughout the movement.

3. As you pull the bar upward focus on leading with the elbows and pulling the shoulder blades down and back. Create a big chest in the finish position.

4. The upper arms should be at close to a 45-degree angle to the torso through the movement.

5. Once the bar touches your torso, follow the same path back down until the arms are completely straight.

VARIATION EXECUTION

If performing the bent-over row with a single arm, keep the torso rigid to fight rotation.

COMMON FAULTS

- *Rounding the back.*
  - Focus on keeping the back as stiff as possible once you are in the beginning position.
  - Focus on maintaining whole-foot pressure, maybe even favoring the heels a bit more.
  - Try to push your hips backward to get into the bent-over position.
- *Cheating, jerking, and moving the torso incorrectly.*
  - Focus on moving in a controlled manner. Do not use momentum or other motion to assist you. The only things that should move are the dumbbells and your arms.
  - Keep your forearms vertical when the bar touches your torso.

INVERTED ROW

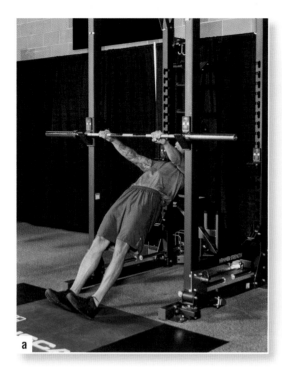
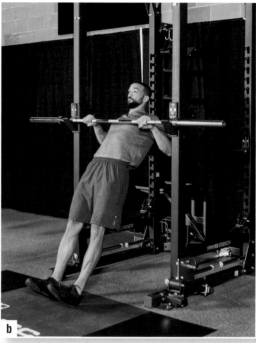

SETUP

1. Start by adjusting the placement of the bar so that it is slightly more than an arm's length from the floor. (You can place it further from the floor if this setup makes it too difficult to perform all prescribed repetitions.)

2. To help hold your feet in place you can put a bench, box, or heavy dumbbell at the base of your feet.

3. Drive your heels into the floor, lean your torso back, and extend your hips, creating an inverted push-up position *(a)*.

4. With a neutral to slightly rounded (not rounded) spine, keep a straight line from your head through your shoulders, hips, knees, and ankles.

5. If this position proves to be too difficult, you can adjust the bar as previously mentioned or flex your knees to 90 degrees.

VARIATION SETUP

You can use a suspension trainer in place of a fixed bar. Start seated on the ground with your hips directly under the anchor point of the trainer and your legs straight. The top of your head should point toward the closed end of the J-hook.

EXECUTION

1. Keep your torso tight and your body rigid, maintaining a straight line from your head through your shoulders, hips, knees, and ankles throughout the entire range of motion.

2. Pull your body up toward the bar while driving the shoulder blades down and back. Create a big chest in the finish position *(b)*.

3. Your upper arms should travel in a 45-degree angle to your torso, stopping when your torso touches the bar.

4. In this top position your hands should be in the same place they would be when the bar touches your torso during bench press.

5. Make a controlled descent back down to the beginning position.

VARIATION EXECUTION

Complete the movement the same way you would if using a fixed bar.

COMMON FAULTS

- *Not maintaining a straight line from your head through your shoulders, hips, knees, and ankles.*
  - ☐ Focus on keeping the entire body rigid, moving as one unit, throughout the movement.
  - ☐ Reexamine your hip or pelvis position. Often the hips will sag if the angle makes the exercise too difficult or because of a lack of focus on keeping the hips engaged to maintain form. If the former, adjust the bar to a better position.
- *The bar is touching too high on the torso.*
  - ☐ Reexamine the intent to contact the bar at a place similar to where the bar touches your torso during a bench press.
  - ☐ Slide backward, bringing your feet a little close to the bar.

PRONE ROW

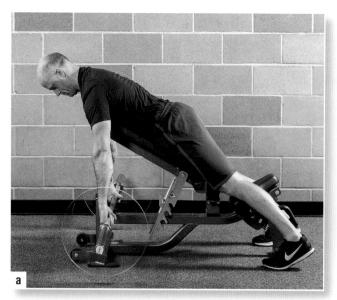
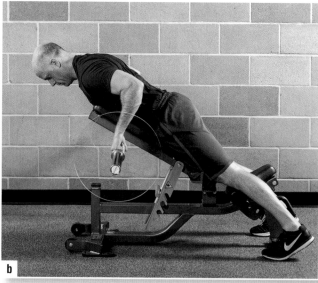

SETUP

1. Set the bench to an incline of about 30 to 45 degrees.

2. Lie prone (face down) on the bench, with the chest and stomach resting on the bench and the head in a neutral position.

3. Position yourself on the bench so that the barbell does not rest on or touch the floor or the bench.

4. Hold the barbell at arm's length with the arms extended toward the floor *(a)*.

5. Plant the feet on the floor for stability.

VARIATION SETUP

Set up dumbbells or kettlebells in a similar position as the barbell.

EXECUTION

1. Pull the barbell up toward a place between the bottom of your chest and the bottom of your rib cage, just outside your torso and the bench.

2. The chest should stay in contact with the bench the entire time.

3. As you pull the barbell up, focus on leading with the elbows and pulling the shoulder blades down and back. Create a big chest in the finish position *(b)*.

4. The upper arms should be at close to a 45-degree angle to the torso through the movement.

5. Once the barbell is in line with your torso, follow the same path back down until the arms are completely straight.

VARIATION EXECUTION

If performing the prone row with a barbell, it will touch the bottom of the bench at the top of each repetition. If performing the exercise with dumbbells or kettlebells, they can be lifted with alternating arms while keeping the body stable on the bench.

COMMON FAULT

- *Cheating, jerking, and moving the torso incorrectly.* Focus on controlling your movement. Do not use momentum or other motion to assist you. The only body part that should move are your arms.

BICEPS CURL

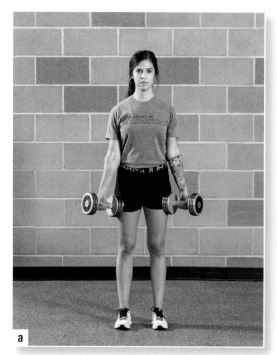
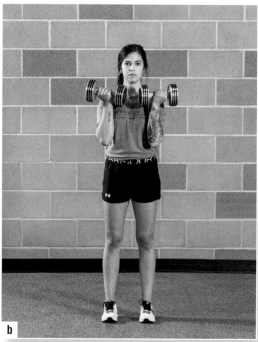

SETUP

1. Hold a dumbbell in each hand and stand with your feet shoulder-width apart.

2. The dumbbells should be next to your thighs or just slightly in front of them.

3. The upper arms should be fixed to your torso and angled forward about 10 degrees away from perpendicular to the floor *(a)*.

4. Your palms should be facing away from your body.

VARIATION SETUP

1. If using a band, loop one end of the band under your feet and stand on it while holding the other end of the band in your hands, keeping in mind the resistance level will increase at the top of the curl.

2. If using a suspension trainer, set up with straight arms, your body in a straight line, and your heels dug into the ground as a pivot point *(c)*.

EXECUTION

1. Pull or raise the dumbbells in an upward-arching fashion toward your face.

2. Continue this motion until the dumbbells touch your shoulders or your elbows cannot flex any further *(b)*.

3. Keep your torso rigid with minimal to no movement of the upper arms.

4. Once the dumbbells touch your shoulders or you cannot flex your elbows any further, return the dumbbells to the beginning position, following the same path back down.

VARIATION EXECUTION

If using a suspension trainer, flex the elbows to curl the body toward the handles without letting the elbows drop *(d)*.

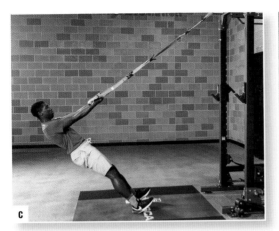
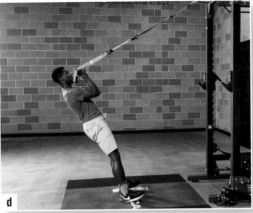

COMMON FAULT

- *Adding movement at the hips or torso.* The hips and torso should remain in a fixed position. Any additional movement is most likely the result of a weight that is too heavy. Reduce the weight and keep the repetitions clean.

REAR DELTOID RAISE

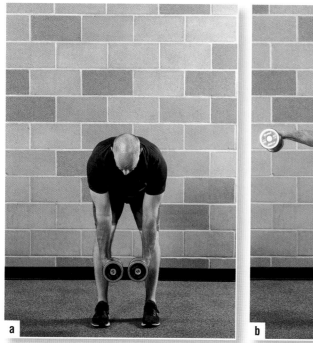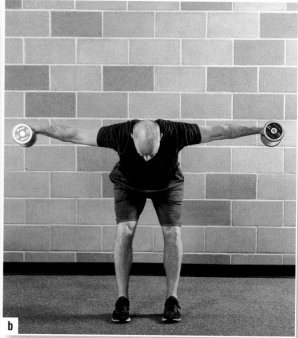

SETUP

1. Hold a dumbbell in each hand, and stand with your feet shoulder-width apart or slightly wider.

2. Get into a bent-over position by pushing your hips backward and allowing the knees to flex slightly.

3. The back should be in a neutral to slightly arched (not rounded) position and should be as close to parallel to the floor as possible while maintaining this neutral position.

4. The head is in a neutral position that is in line with your spine.

5. In this bent-over position your arms should be almost straight with your hands and dumbbells directly under your shoulders *(a)*.

VARIATION SETUP

If using a suspension trainer, start the movement in a fairly upright position with a neutral grip as though you are about to start an extremely easy inverted row.

EXECUTION

1. Raise the dumbbells outward, keeping the elbow joint fixed.

2. Continue to raise the dumbbells until your elbows are in line with your shoulders *(b)*.

3. Follow the same path down to the starting position, controlling the descent.

VARIATION EXECUTION

If using a suspension trainer, open the arms in the same fashion as described above until your body forms a T. Reverse the movement under control to return to the beginning position. Maintain tension on the straps throughout the entire movement.

COMMON FAULTS

- *Rounding the back.*
  - □ Focus on keeping the back as stiff as possible once you are in the initial position.
  - □ In the setup be sure to push your hip back to get into the bent-over position.
- *Cheating, jerking, and moving the torso incorrectly.* Focus on moving in a controlled manner. Do not use momentum or other motion to assist you. The only things that should move are the dumbbells and your arms.

FACEPULL

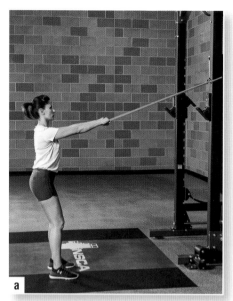 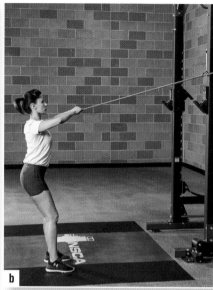 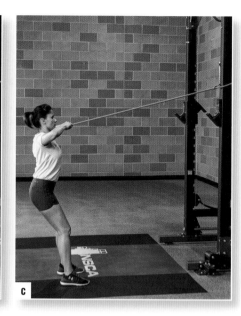

SETUP

1. If possible, align the cable so that the handle connection point is between chin height and head height.

2. Attach a rope handle or similar style handle to the cable.

3. Facing the machine, grab the handle with an overhand grip (palms toward the floor).

4. Step back from the machine until your arms are fully extended out in front of you and there is no slack on the cable.

5. Your arms should be at or above parallel to the floor and your torso perpendicular to slightly leaned back.

VARIATION SETUP

1. If using a band, the setup is like that of the cable, but you might grasp the band in the absence of a handle *(a)*.

2. If using a suspension trainer, the setup like that of an inverted row exercise but at a more upright angle.

EXECUTION

1. Pull the handle toward your face, leading with the elbows.

2. The elbows should travel upward slightly (no higher than your eyebrows) and back as far as your range of motion comfortably allows *(b)*.

3. As you pull and your hands travel to your face, your middle fingers should be about eyebrow height as they graze your skin *(c)*.

4. Once your elbows are as far back as they can comfortably go and your middle fingers travel to or past your eyebrows, follow the same path back to the beginning position.

VARIATION EXECUTION

If using a suspension trainer, in place of pulling the cable or band toward you, keep your body in a straight line and use the same execution steps as above to pull your face toward the handles.

COMMON FAULTS

- *Going too fast.* Control the entire motion.

- *Using momentum.* Your torso should be perpendicular to the floor or just slightly leaned back. Once you find your beginning position the torso should remain still. If movement is needed from a portion of your body besides your arm to execute the movement, reduce the weight.

- *Dropping the elbows on the return to the beginning position.* Focus on keeping the elbows about eyebrow height for as long as you can. As your elbows extend they will have to lower, but do not allow it to happen any sooner. You need the return action to mirror the pull.

HAMMER CURL

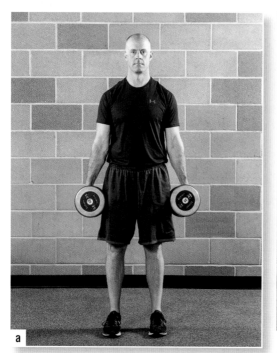 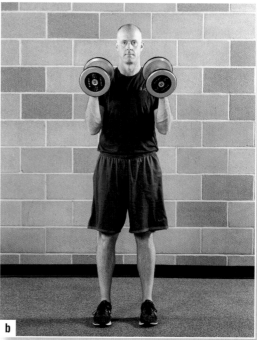

SETUP

1. Hold a dumbbell in each hand with your palms facing inward, and stand with your feet shoulder-width apart.
2. The dumbbells should be just outside of each respective thigh *(a)*.

EXECUTION

1. Pull or raise the dumbbells in an upward-arching fashion toward your face.
2. Continue this motion until the dumbbells touch your shoulders or your elbows cannot flex any further *(b)*.
3. Keep your torso rigid with minimal to no movement of the upper arms.
4. Once the dumbbells touch your shoulders or you cannot flex your elbows any further, return the dumbbells to the starting position following the same path back down.

COMMON FAULT

■ *Adding movement at the hips or torso.* The hips and torso should remain in a fixed position. Any additional movement is most likely the result of a weight that is too heavy. Reduce the weight and keep the repetitions clean.

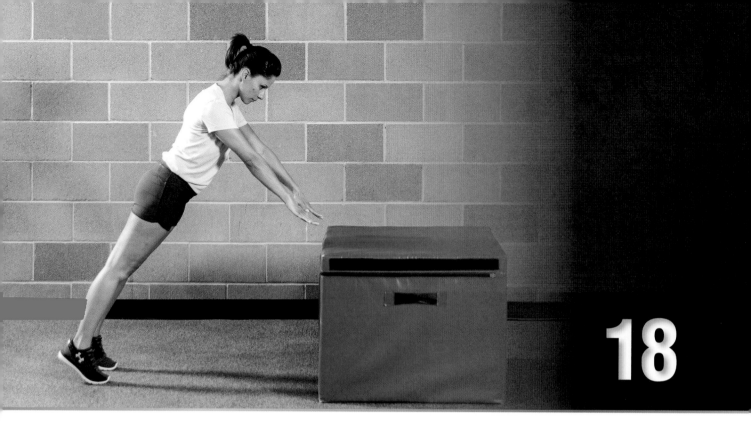

18

Upper Body Pushing Exercises

Upper body pushing exercises build strength and endurance for the chest, triceps, and shoulders. This strength and endurance supports the demands of the HRP event. In the absence of specific equipment, push-ups travel extremely well and are easy to load with bands, weight plates, a body armor, and even manual resistance.

Upper Body Pushing Exercises Finder

ALTERNATIVE UPPER BODY PUSHING EXERCISES

The upper body pushing exercises included in the chapter 12 programs are the preferred exercises as they relate to the ACFT. If you do not have the needed equipment to do a preferred exercise, you will need to choose an alternative exercise. Go to table 18.1 and find the exercise you need to replace along the top row. (The name will not include the piece of equipment being used.) Next, find the equipment options to which you have access along the left-hand column. Your alternative exercise options are where the column of the exercise you are replacing intersects the rows of the types of equipment to which you have access. Choose the option that best mimics the position, movement, and resistance level of the preferred exercise in the chapter 12 programs. Note that not every type of equipment supports an alternative exercise, but at least one body weight replacement exists for every exercise, so there is no excuse to entirely omit a programmed exercise.

Table 18.1   Alternative Upper Body Pushing Exercises

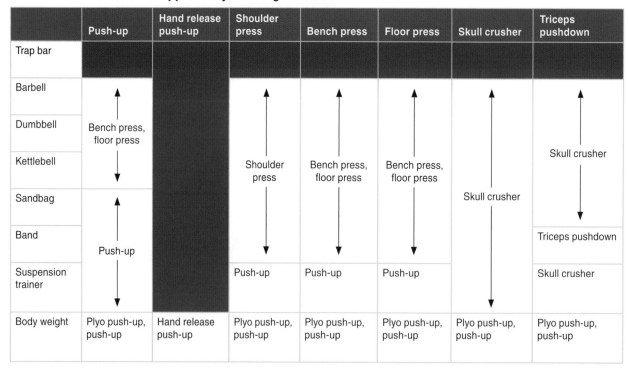

	Push-up	Hand release push-up	Shoulder press	Bench press	Floor press	Skull crusher	Triceps pushdown
Trap bar							
Barbell			↑	↑	↑	↑	↑
Dumbbell	Bench press, floor press ↑↓						
Kettlebell			Shoulder press	Bench press, floor press	Bench press, floor press		Skull crusher
Sandbag	Push-up ↑↓					Skull crusher	
Band							Triceps pushdown ↓
Suspension trainer			Push-up	Push-up	Push-up		Skull crusher
Body weight	Plyo push-up, push-up	Hand release push-up	Plyo push-up, push-up	Plyo push-up, push-up	Plyo push-up, push-up	Plyo push-up, push-up	Plyo push-up, push-up

PUSH-UP

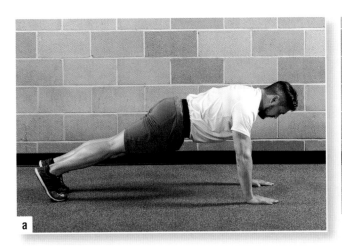
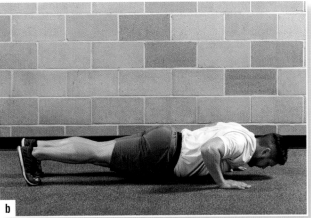

SETUP

1. Lie face down in a prone position.
2. Place your hands underneath your shoulders with whole-hand pressure on the floor.
3. Place your feet hip-width apart with pressure into the floor through the balls of your feet.
4. Form a straight line from your head through your shoulders, hips, knees, and ankles *(a)*.

VARIATION SETUP

1. To add weight, place weight on the upper back or wear a weighted vest.
2. If using a suspension trainer, place your hands in the handles.
3. If using a band, wrap the band around your upper back (where the weight would be placed) and put your hands through each end of the loop, pinning the band against the floor *(c)*.
4. If performing with a single arm, incline the upper body to an angle that reduces the load as much as needed.
5. If performing on a pair dumbbells, position them under the shoulders and use a fully-closed grip on the handles.

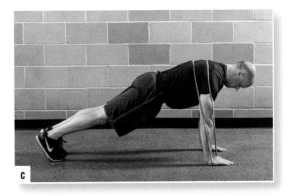

EXECUTION

1. Keep your torso tight and your body rigid, maintaining a straight line from your head through your shoulders, hips, knees, and ankles throughout the entire range of motion.
2. Lower your body until your chest touches the floor.
3. In the bottom position your upper arm should be at a 45-degree angle to your torso with your elbows close to directly over your wrists *(b)*.
4. Push away from the floor, fully extending your arms, until you are back to the beginning position.

VARIATION EXECUTION

1. Adjust the band as needed to increase or decrease resistance.

2. Incline the feet or add resistance to make the suspension trainer variation more difficult.

3. If performing with a single arm, resist rotation to keep your body level, and adjust the angle as needed to decrease or increase resistance.

4. If performing on a pair dumbbells, lower your body the extra distance to the floor.

COMMON FAULTS

- *Elbows flaring out.*
  - Maintain a 45-degree angle of the upper arm in relation to the torso.
  - Be aware of the triceps' contribution to the movement.
- *Not maintaining a straight line from the head through your shoulders, hips, knees, and ankles.*
  - Reexamine the intent to keep the entire body rigid, moving as one unit, throughout the movement.
  - Focus on your hip or pelvis position. Often, they tilt in a manner that causes an arch in the back and the abdominals to lose tension. If this is the case, tilt them by engaging your glutes. (Think of a scared dog tucking its tail.)
- *Training through repetitions even when you cannot maintain proper position and execution.* Reduce the weight or the repetitions.

HAND RELEASE PUSH-UP

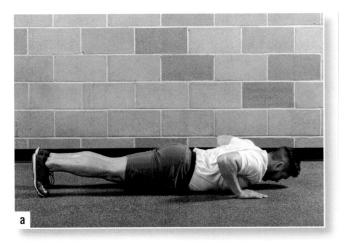

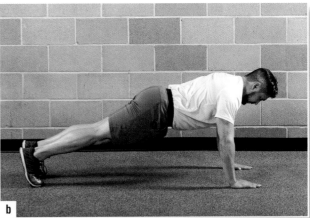

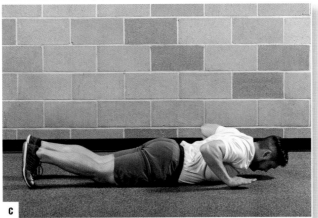

SETUP

1. Lie face down in a prone position.
2. The chest, hips, and thighs (but not head) should be in contact with the ground.
3. Place your hands underneath your shoulders, with the index finger inside the broadest part of your shoulders, with whole-hand pressure on the floor.
4. The feet are no more than a boot's width apart.
5. Form a straight line from your head through your shoulders, hips, knees, and ankles *(a)*.

EXECUTION

1. Keep your torso tight and your body rigid, maintaining a straight line from your head through your shoulders, hips, knees, and ankles throughout the entire range of motion.
2. Push away from the floor, fully extending your arms *(b)*.
3. Lower your body until your chest, hips, and thighs (but not head) are in contact with the floor.
4. Bring your hands back under your shoulders, placing them just above the beginning position *(c)*.
5. Repeat the process for the prescribed number of repetitions.

COMMON FAULTS

- *Elbows flaring out.*
  - ☐ Maintain a 45-degree angle of the upper arm in relation to the torso.
  - ☐ Be aware of the triceps' contribution to the movement.
- *Not maintaining a straight line from the head through your shoulders, hips, knees, and ankles.*
  - ☐ Reexamine the intent to keep the entire body rigid, moving as one unit, throughout the movement.
  - ☐ Focus on your hip or pelvis position. Often, they tilt in a manner that causes an arch in the back or the abdominals to lose tension. If this is the case, tilt them by engaging your glutes. (Think of a scared dog tucking its tail.)
- *Training through repetitions even when you cannot maintain proper position and execution.* Reduce repetitions in each set.

SHOULDER PRESS

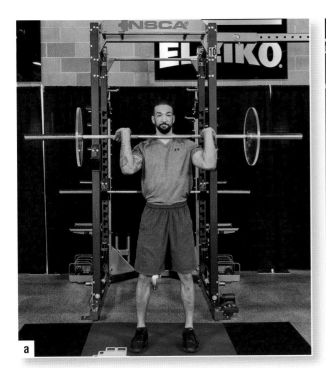
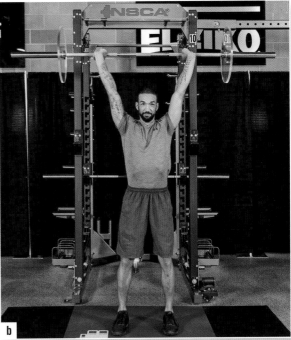

SETUP

1. Stand with your feet flat on the floor, hip to shoulder width apart.

2. Extend the hips and knees, and tense the muscles of the lower body. Maintain a neutral to slightly arched (not rounded) spine.

3. Activate the glutes to ensure proper hip and pelvis position and prevent lower back discomfort.

4. The grip is in line with or slightly wider than shoulder width.

5. Maintain a neutral wrist position (unlike what is seen in the photos).

6. The bar should touch the top of the shoulders *(a)*.

VARIATION SETUP

1. If using dumbbells or kettlebells, you can start with them either in front of and close to the chest or with the arms in a similar position as the barbell setup.

2. If using a band, loop the band under the feet and through the hands, starting from the same position as the barbell shoulder press.

EXECUTION

1. Aside from the bar position, maintain the initial setup throughout the movement.

2. The head and chin slide back (give yourself a double chin) to make way for the vertical bar path.

3. Press the bar overhead until the arms are fully extended *(b)*.

4. The bar finishes directly over the spine.

5. Follow the same bar path back down to the shoulders, and repeat for prescribed number of repetitions.

VARIATION EXECUTION

If performing with a single arm, keep the torso rigid and do not let the unilaterally loaded weight cause your body to sway to one side.

COMMON FAULT

- *Pressing the bar in front of your head instead of over your head.* Drive the bar straight up and slightly back so that it ends up directly over your spine when the arms are fully extended.

BENCH PRESS

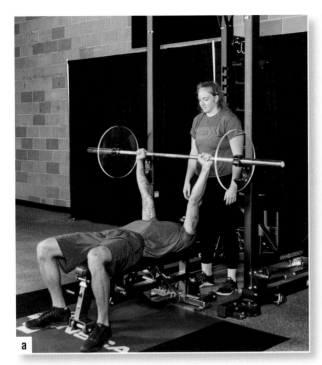
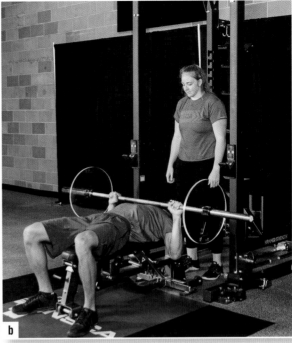

SETUP

1. Position yourself on the bench so the bar is aligned over your forehead.

2. Either the balls of your feet or the entire foot should be flat on the ground.

3. The feet should also be aligned so your knees are lower than your hips. Depending on preference and mobility your feet might be underneath you or extended in front of you.

4. The hips and glutes should be engaged and always in contact with the bench.

5. The shoulder blades should be pulled down and back, creating tension and a stable base from which to press.

6. The head should remain in contact with the bench.

7. Grip the bar so the forearms are vertical when the bar touches the torso and the upper arms are at a 45-degree angle relative to the torso.

VARIATION SETUP

1. If using dumbbells or kettlebells, the setup is similar, but hold weights at chest height and lie back under control to get into the beginning position. If using a spotter, he or she should spot the wrists or the inside of the weight itself. Spotting the elbows or outside of the weight can cause it to collapse inward.

2. If using a band, wrap the band underneath the bench or your back to secure it. Loop each end through your hands, choking up as much as needed to adjust resistance.

3. You can also incline the bench to about 45 degrees.

4. If using a neutral grip, face the palms toward each other and keep the elbows tight to your sides.

EXECUTION

1. It is preferable to lift off from the rack and position the bar in a comfortable and stable position over your shoulders *(a)*.

2. Lower the bar to your torso at a point where the forearms are vertical and the upper arms are at a 45-degree angle.

3. Touch the bar to the torso, but do not bounce it off your torso *(b)*.

4. Press the bar up and back slightly to the original beginning position over your shoulders.

VARIATION EXECUTION

1. If performing with a single arm, resist rotation by staying engaged through your abdominals and driving your legs aggressively into the ground.

2. If using a neutral grip, keep the palms facing each other and elbows tight to your sides throughout the movement.

COMMON FAULTS

■ *Hips coming off the bench.* Reexamine the alignment of your knees in relation to your hips, remembering the knees should be lower. If they are not, adjust your feet accordingly. You want to create tension, not lift, by using your feet.

■ *Bouncing the bar off your chest.* Control the bar on the descent. If you cannot control it, reduce the weight.

■ *Touching too low or too high on the torso.* Focus on keeping the forearms vertical when the bar touches your torso.

■ *Pressing the bar away or straight up.* Reexamine your effort to drive the bar up and back simultaneously.

■ *Not grounding the feet on the floor.* Put some bumper plates underneath your feet. Benches are not one-size-fits-all.

FLOOR PRESS

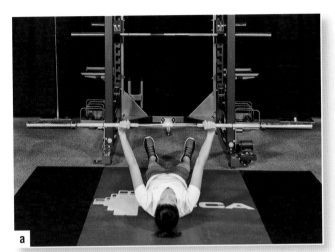
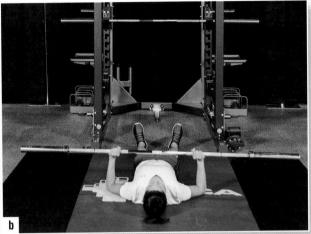

SETUP

1. Position yourself on the floor so the bar is aligned over your forehead.

2. Knees should be flexed to about 90 degrees, much like a sit-up beginning position except wider for a better base of support. The feet should be on the ground with the entire foot laid flat. As an alternative, the legs can lie flat with the toes pointed up (as seen in the photos).

3. The hips and glutes should be engaged and always in contact with the floor.

4. The shoulder blades should be pulled down and back, creating tension and a stable base from which to press.

5. Head should remain in contact with the floor.

6. Grip the bar so the forearms are vertical when the bar touches the torso and the upper arms are at a 45-degree angle relative to the torso (check this before you start the exercise).

VARIATION SETUP

1. If using dumbbells or kettlebells, the setup is similar, but hold the weights at chest height and lie back under control to get into the beginning position. If using a spotter, he or she should spot the wrists or the inside of the weight itself. Spotting the elbows or outside of the weight can cause it to collapse inward.

2. If using a band, wrap the band underneath your back to secure it. Loop each end through your hands, choking up as much as needed to adjust resistance.

EXECUTION

1. Position the bar in a comfortable and stable position over your shoulders *(a)*.

2. Lower the bar to your torso at a point where the forearms are vertical and the upper arms are at a 45-degree angle relative to the torso.

3. Your elbows will contact the floor lightly prior to the bar reaching your torso *(b)*.

4. Press the bar up and back slightly to the original beginning position over your shoulders.

COMMON FAULTS

- *Bouncing your elbows off the floor.* Control the bar on the descent. If you cannot control it, reduce the weight.

- *Pressing the bar away or straight up.* Reexamine your effort to drive the bar up and back simultaneously.

PLYO PUSH-UP

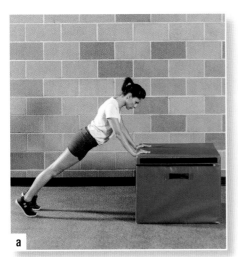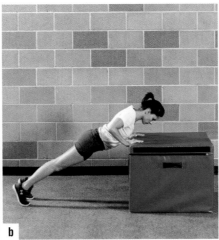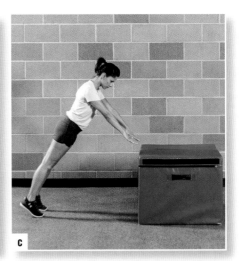

a   b   c

SETUP

1. Lie face down in a prone position on the box edge.
2. Place your hands underneath your shoulders with your elbows extended and whole-hand pressure on the box.
3. Feet should be hip-width apart with pressure into the floor through the balls of your feet.
4. Keep a straight line from your head through your shoulders, hips, knees, and ankles.

EXECUTION

1. Keep your torso tight and your body rigid, maintaining a straight line from your head through your shoulders, hips, knees, and ankles throughout the entire range of motion *(a)*.
2. Allow your body to lower toward the box as fast as you can control, instantly reversing the action before your chest touches the box. (If you were able to freeze the action in the bottom position, your upper arm should be at a 45-degree angle to your torso with your elbows directly over your wrists *[b]*.)
3. That instant reversal of the action should continue with the intent of pushing the box away as fast as possible.
4. This forceful intent should continue through full extension of the arms, launching your torso, arms, and hands off the box into the air *(c)*.
5. Once gravity takes over, prepare to contact the box by flexing the elbows as the hands touch the box.
6. Once the hands touch the box, proceed back to step 2 and continue for the prescribed number of repetitions.

COMMON FAULTS

- *Elbows flaring out.*
  - ☐ Maintain a 45-degree angle of the upper arms in relation to the torso.
  - ☐ Be aware of the triceps' contribution to the movement.

■ *Not maintaining a straight line from the head through your shoulders, hips, knees, and ankles.*
  - Reexamine the intent to keep the entire body rigid, moving as one unit, throughout the movement.
  - Focus on your hip or pelvis position. Often, they tilt in a manner that causes an arch in the back or for the abdominals to lose tension. If this is the case, tilt them by engaging your glutes. (Think of a scared dog tucking its tail.)

■ *Training through repetitions even if you cannot maintain proper position and execution.*
  - Reduce the intensity by resting your knees on the floor if you don't use a box for the exercise.
  - Reduce the intensity by moving your hands from the floor to an elevated object such as a bench, stairs, or a box (as seen in the photos).

SKULL CRUSHER

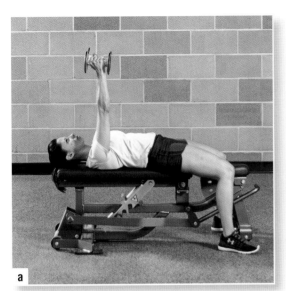
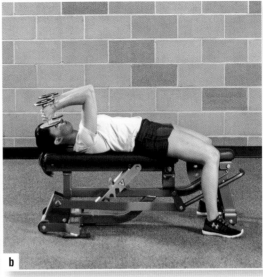

SETUP

1. Position yourself on the bench so that your head, shoulders, and hips are all comfortably in contact with the bench.

2. Either the balls of your feet or the entire foot should be flat on the floor.

3. The hips or glutes should be engaged and always in contact with the bench.

4. The head should remain in contact with the bench.

5. Position the dumbbells directly over the shoulders with the arms fully extended and the palms facing each other *(a)*.

VARIATION SETUP

1. In the absence of a bench, you can set up similarly on the floor.

2. If using a band, loop it under your back or under the bench and grab each end, choking up as much as needed to adjust the resistance.

3. If using a suspension trainer, begin in the top of a push-up position but with a much less aggressive angle *(c)*.

EXECUTION

1. Maintaining the hand position or neutral grip (palms facing each other), allow your upper arms to slightly travel toward your head, creating about a 5-degree angle from the perpendicular starting position.

2. Keeping your upper arms in this position throughout the range of motion, allow your hands to move toward your head or slightly over, with the movement occurring at the elbow joint alone *(b)*.

3. As the dumbbells approach your head, they should travel to their respective sides of the head, allowing greater range of motion.

4. Once the forearms approach a position parallel to the floor, reverse the action, following the same path back to the starting point.

VARIATION EXECUTION

If using a suspension trainer, flex your elbows to lower your forehead to the handles while maintaining a straight line from your head to your heels *(c)*. Extend your elbows to return to the start position *(d)*.

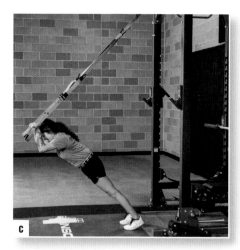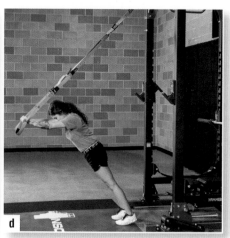

COMMON FAULT

- *Allowing the upper arms to move.* Keep the upper arms still throughout the range of motion. Often, they move because too much weight is being used. If this is the case, reduce the weight.

TRICEPS PUSHDOWN

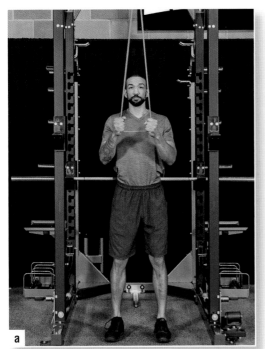
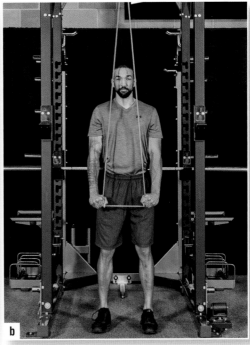

SETUP

1. Loop a band around a pull-up bar or something stable at a similar height.

2. Grab the band at the lowest point, facing away from the pull-up bar.

3. Take a step or two away from the pull-up bar, allowing your arms and the band to go up close to your head. Your upper arms are fully extended and in line with your head and spine.

EXECUTION

1. Allow the band to pull your hands back toward the pull-up bar, keeping your upper arms fixed in alignment with your head and spine *(a)*.

2. Once your hands reach the furthest back position that is comfortably achieved without any upper arm movement, return them to the starting position by extending the elbows *(b)*.

3. Perform this action in a controlled manner for the first number of prescribed repetitions. Your upper arms are fully extended and in line with your head and spine.

4. Once those repetitions are completed, immediately, without rest, turn and face the pull-up bar, and step toward it until you are directly underneath it or just slightly in front of it. You may also need to flex your knees slightly to get the desired tension on the band.

5. The band should now be in front of you and your arms should be flexed as much as possible with your hands near shoulder height.

6. In this position, extend and flex your elbows as quickly as you can, allowing for a full range of motion with minimal to no movement of the upper arms.

COMMON FAULT

■ *Turning it into a decline press–type of movement.* Keep the elbows tight to your side; do not let them flare out. Keep the upper arms fixed with minimal to no movement throughout the range of motion.

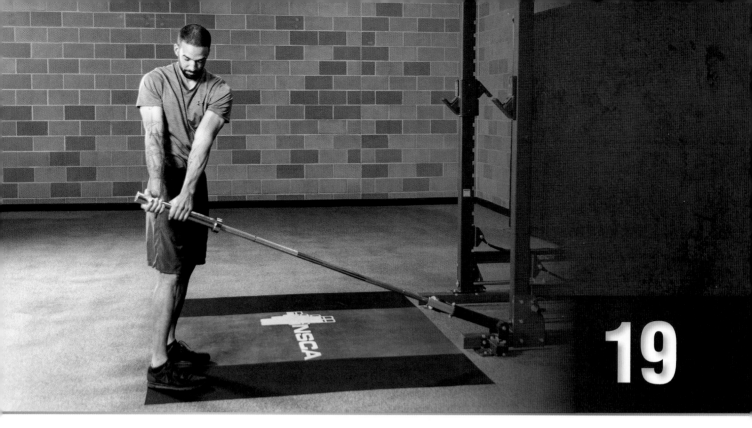

Trunk Exercises

For the purposes of this book, trunk exercises primarily target the abdominal muscles by creating or resisting movement in all planes. They have obvious carryover to the LTK event but quietly contribute to every ACFT event in some way. The trunk muscles generate and resist force, making them a vital component of explosive movements and an undeniable factor in the prevention of injuries.

Trunk Exercises Finder

ALTERNATIVE TRUNK EXERCISES

The trunk exercises included in the chapter 12 programs are the preferred exercises as they relate to the ACFT. If you do not have the equipment to do a preferred exercise, you will need to choose an alternative exercise. Go to table 19.1 and find the exercise you need to replace along the top row. (The name will not include the piece of equipment being used.) Next, find the equipment options to which you have access in the left column. Your alternative exercise options are where the column of the exercise you are replacing intersects the rows of the types of equipment to which you have access. Choose the option that best mimics the position, movement, and resistance level of the preferred exercise in the chapter 12 programs. Note that not every type of equipment supports an alternative exercise, but at least one body weight replacement exists for every exercise, so there is no excuse to entirely omit a programmed exercise.

Table 19.1 Alternative Trunk Exercises*

	Hanging knee raise	Ab rollout	Landmine twist	Pallof press	Half kneeling chop and lift	Stir the pot	Roman side crunch	Body saw	Side bend	Farmer walk
Trap bar										Farmer walk
Barbell		Ab rollout	Landmine twist		Landmine twist	Ab rollout		Ab rollout		
Dumbbell										Farmer walk
Kettlebell					Half kneeling chop and lift		Side bend		Side bend	
Sandbag										
Band										
Suspension trainer		Ab rollout				Stir the pot		Ab rollout		
Body weight	Reverse crunch	Front plank, eccentric dragon flag	Lying trunk twist	Single-arm plank, single-leg plank	Lying trunk twist	Front plank	Side plank (for reps)	Front plank	Side plank (for reps)	Front plank

*The front plank, side plank, reverse crunch, sit-up, deadbug, eccentric dragon flag, leg tuck, and lying trunk twist are originally bodyweight exercises and, therefore, they do not have any suggested non-bodyweight alternatives.

FRONT PLANK

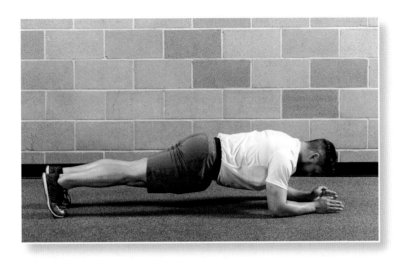

SETUP

1. Lie in the prone position (face down) with your elbows directly under your shoulders, your arms parallel to each other, your toes tucked, and your neck neutral. (Making a double chin helps maintain a neutral neck.)

2. When weighted, place weight across the lower back or wear a weighted vest.

VARIATION SETUP

If performing the front plank with a single-arm or a single-leg, get into the same beginning position as the front plank.

EXECUTION

1. Raise your body off the floor.

2. Maintain a straight line from your head through your heels.

3. Be active in this position by driving your legs straight, squeezing your butt, pushing your elbows into the floor, and tucking your tail so that you feel constant tension in your abdominals.

VARIATION EXECUTION

If performing the single-arm front plank, lift one hand and point the arm forward; if performing the single-leg front plank, lift one foot and point the leg backward. For either variation, squeeze your butt to straighten your hips and tighten your torso to fight rotation. Switch to the other arm or leg for the next set, or alternate the arms or legs with each repetition.

COMMON FAULTS

- *Hips sagging.* Pull your hips off the floor so that your body is in a straight line and you feel the exercise in the front of your body and not your lower back.

- *Hips going too high.* Squeeze your butt to straighten your hips and keep a straight line from your head to your heels. A partner can help improve your positional awareness by providing verbal feedback.

SIDE PLANK

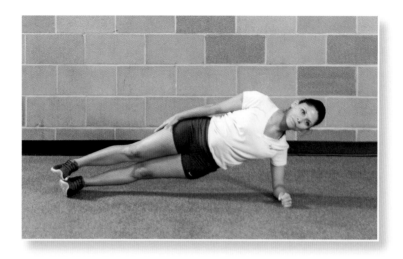

SETUP

1. Lie on your side with your legs stacked one on top of the other and your bottom elbow under your shoulder.

2. Let the top arm rest along the side of your body like the position of attention, and stare straight ahead.

EXECUTION

1. Drive your hips up off the ground until your body forms a straight line from the head to the heel.

2. Continue to push into the ground through your elbow and squeeze your butt.

3. Hold this position for the prescribed amount of time.

4. These can also be done for repetitions as a substitute for the dumbbell side bend or Roman side crunch.

COMMON FAULTS

■ *Sitting back into the hips.* Squeeze your butt to get your hips to a neutral position.

■ *Looking down.* Look straight ahead and make a double chin to help keep your neck neutral.

REVERSE CRUNCH

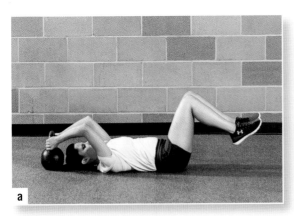
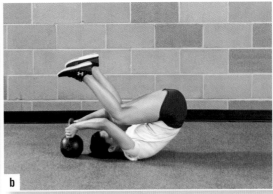

SETUP

1. Lie down with your back on the floor.

2. Bring your legs up so that your hips and knees are at a 90-degree angle, making sure your lower back is in contact with the floor *(a)*.

3. If possible, position a kettlebell, frame of a rack, or a heavy item of support about 6 inches (15 cm) away from the top of your head. If not, place your fingers tips on the side of your head.

4. The elbows should be bent at close to a 90-degree angle.

EXECUTION

1. Begin by engaging the abdominals and pushing the low back further into the floor.

2. Using the tension created by engaging your abdominals, increase this engagement, causing the pelvis and, subsequently, the entire lower body to curl toward your head.

3. Imagine each individual vertebra flexing sequentially from the pelvis toward the head as the lower body travels toward your elbows as one fixed unit.

4. Continue this motion until your knees touch your elbows or you cannot curl or crunch any further *(b)*.

5. Once you hit your specific end position, reverse the action, controlling the descent back through the same path followed on the way up.

COMMON FAULTS

■ *Allowing the hips to extend past a 90-degree angle.* Reexamine the controlled descent and the goal of stopping the movement when the hips return to their original 90-degree angle. Going past that can also result in lower back discomfort.

■ *Using momentum to initiate the movement.* Perform the movement in a controlled manner on both the way up and the way down by re-examining the starting point of each repetition, making sure the hips are not going past that 90-degree beginning position on the way down.

SIT-UP

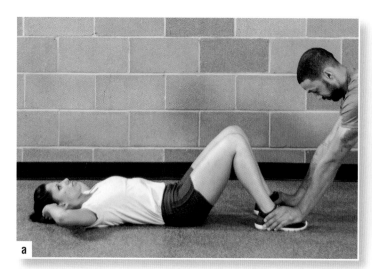
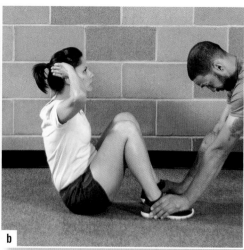

SETUP

1. Lie on the ground with your feet near your butt so that your knees form a 90-degree angle or less.

2. Place your hands adjacent to your head or your arms across your chest to avoid straining your neck.

3. Keep the hips, knees, and feet in line and the feet anchored on the floor. (You can also place them underneath something like a sit-up bar or partner's hands *[a]*.)

EXECUTION

1. Raise your back off the floor until your spine is perpendicular or past perpendicular to the floor *(b)*.

2. Lower your back down to the starting position without losing tension in your abdominals.

COMMON FAULT

■ *Not controlling the range of motion.* Build proper abdominal and hip flexor function by maintaining control throughout the exercise.

HANGING KNEE RAISE

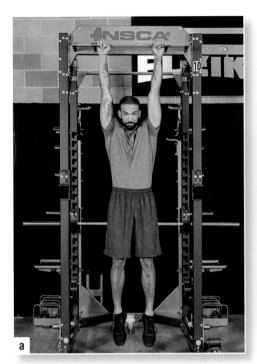 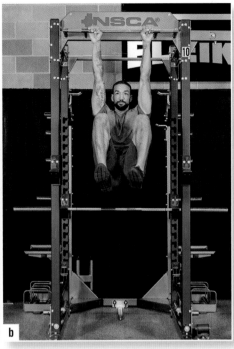

SETUP

1. Hang freely from a pull-up bar with your arms and legs both straight.
2. Grasp the bar with a full grip, wrapping the thumb and fingers from opposite directions *(a)*.

EXECUTION

1. Apply forward and inward pressure to the bar as if breaking it in half.
2. Slowly raise your bent knees toward your elbows without swinging to generate momentum *(b)*.
3. Your knees should pass hip height but can go as high as your elbows so long as you can maintain control.
4. Reverse the movement by lowering your legs under control until your body is hanging in a straight line again.

COMMON FAULTS

- *Swinging to generate momentum.* Slow down and maintain tension in your abdominals throughout the movement. If strength is the issue, consider substituting this exercise with reverse crunches.
- *Bending the elbows.* Keep the arms straight. If restricted shoulder mobility prevents this, look into exercises that increase your range of motion overhead.

DEADBUG

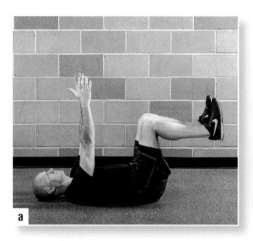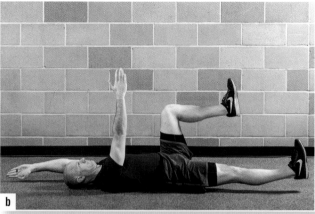

SETUP

1. Lie on your back with your hips and knees at 90 degrees and your arms reaching toward the ceiling.

2. Apply slight pressure into the ground through your lower back to feel your abdominals engage *(a)*.

EXECUTION

1. Simultaneously extend an arm and the opposite leg to lower them toward the floor.

2. Maintain tension in your abdominals by keeping the same pressure between your lower back and the floor.

3. Both the leg and the arm should end as straight and close to the floor as possible without compromising the lower back's position *(b)*.

4. Exhale fully from the extended position and inhale as you return to the beginning position.

5. Repeat the process with the opposite arm and leg, using the same breathing pattern.

6. Common variations are to only alternate the arms (or legs) while keeping the legs (or arms) stationary.

COMMON FAULTS

- *Losing pelvic position (allowing the low back to arch or flex excessively).* Consider decreasing the range of motion or keeping your knee bent as you lower your leg.

- *Bending the overhead arm.* Shorten the range of motion and include exercises to improve shoulder mobility.

AB ROLLOUT

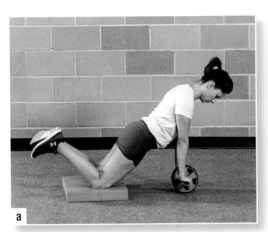 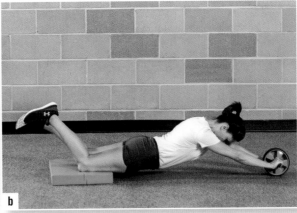

SETUP

1. Start in a tall kneeling position, forming a straight line from your knees through the top of your head.
2. Keep your arms straight and place your hands on the piece of equipment being used (e.g., roller *[a]*, stability ball, suspension trainer).

EXECUTION

1. Fall forward slowly and under control while keeping the arms straight.
2. Maintain a straight line from the knees through the top of the head.
3. Let the arms rise until they are reaching overhead, but keep tension in the abdominals *(b)*.
4. Contract your abdominals to bring the arms back down toward your waist to return to the beginning position.

COMMON FAULT

■ *Breaking at the hips.* Resist the urge to let your butt kick backward, thus losing the straight line from your head to your knees. You should feel tension in your abdominals through the whole exercise. It helps to move slower than you think you want to.

ECCENTRIC DRAGON FLAG

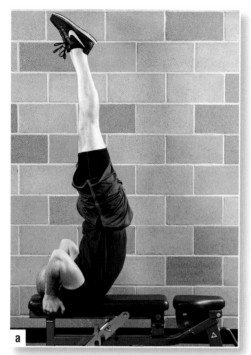 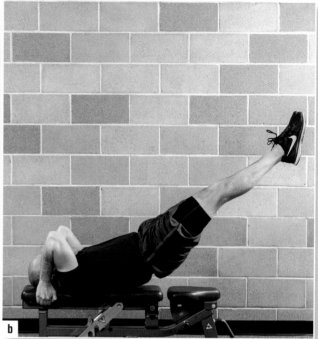

SETUP

1. Lie on your back on the ground or a bench with your legs straight up and hips raised.

2. As much of the back of your body as possible will be off the surface *(a)*.

3. Your hands can hold a fixed object over your head such as a rack, the top of a bench, or someone's legs.

4. This is the starting position for each repetition.

EXECUTION

1. From the beginning position, keep your body as straight as possible, and slowly lower your legs, hips, and back toward the surface *(b)*.

2. Maintain tension in your abdominals throughout the lowering process.

3. Once you lower all the way to the surface, you can bend your legs to return to the beginning position.

COMMON FAULT

■ *Not controlling the entire descent.* Lower at a pace slow enough that you could stop at any point in the movement and hold that position. If the exercise is too difficult for you to keep a straight body while lowering slowly, consider replacing it with a simple front plank or reverse crunches to build more abdominal strength first.

LEG TUCK

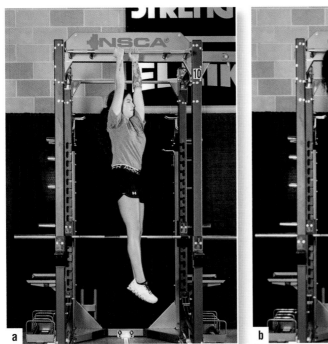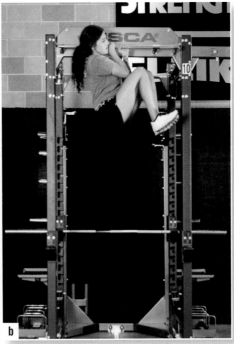

SETUP

1. Hang freely from a pull-up bar with the arms and legs both straight *(a)*.

2. Grasp the bar with a full and mixed or opposing grip so that your palms face each other.

3. Your hands should be fairly close together.

EXECUTION

1. Without swinging to generate momentum, raise your knees toward your elbows until your elbows touch your thighs or knees.

2. Your elbows will bend to about 90 degrees to achieve contact with your legs *(b)*.

3. Return to the beginning position under control and attempt to minimize rotation.

COMMON FAULT

■ *Using momentum to achieve the full range of motion.* This exercise requires substantial upper body pulling and abdominal strength. If you cannot achieve complete repetitions without swinging, consider focusing on developing your pull-up and ab strength independently before combining them.

LYING TRUNK TWIST

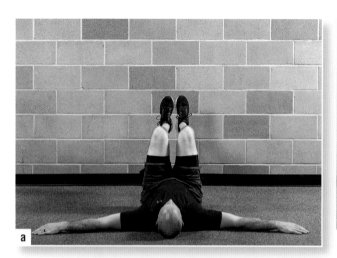
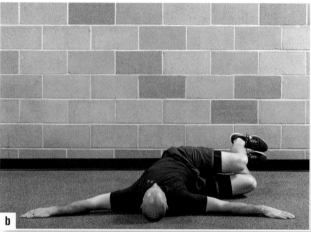

SETUP

1. Lie on your back with your hips and knees at 90 degrees so your feet are in the air *(a)*.

2. Place your arms at your sides, forming about a 45-degree angle between them and your body.

3. Maintain light contact between your lower back and the floor.

EXECUTION

1. With control, let your knees fall toward your side while maintaining the same angle at your hips and knees *(b)*.

2. You will feel tension across your abs as if you are a towel being wrung out.

3. Return to the beginning position to pause briefly before repeating on the opposite side.

COMMON FAULTS

■ *Using momentum.* Slow down to maintain control through the entire range of motion. If you are unable to maintain control, consider replacing this exercise with the Pallof press.

■ *Applying resistance in the wrong direction.* Make sure the resistance is applied at a 90-degree angle from the end of your hands when your arms are extended and not from behind you.

■ *Applying too much resistance.* If you cannot maintain positional integrity and you do not feel the exercise challenging your abs, shuffle your body slightly closer to the anchor point.

LANDMINE TWIST

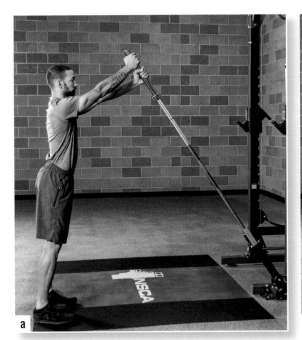
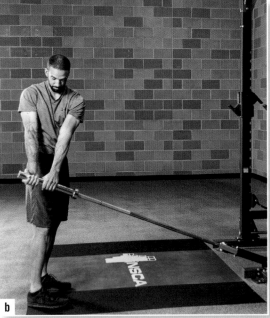

SETUP

1. Secure one end of a barbell into a landmine device or wedge it into the corner of a room, rack, or sandbags. Make sure this end is fixed and will not move.
2. Hold the other end of the barbell straight out in front of your face *(a)*.
3. If additional resistance is desired, load a plate on the top end of the barbell.

EXECUTION

1. Keeping the arms straight, rotate your torso until the bumper plate or barbell touches the side of your hip *(b)*.
2. Rotate in the opposite direction until you touch the opposite hip.
3. Perform the rotation under control.

COMMON FAULT

■ *Generating momentum with your legs.* While this exercise can be performed explosively by loading and exploding through the hips, the intent is to move under control by using the musculature of the torso. If you cannot perform the exercise without using your lower body to generate momentum, consider reducing the weight or substituting an easier rotational ab exercise.

PALLOF PRESS

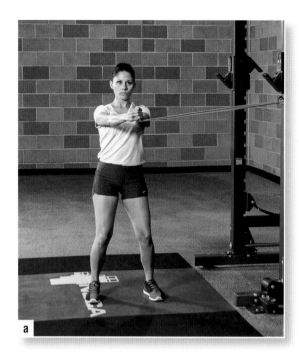
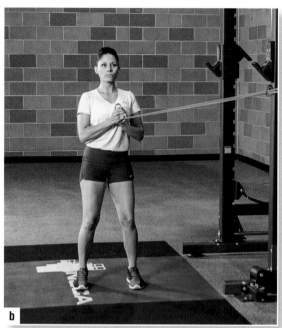

SETUP

1. Grab a band or cable at chest height and step a few feet away from its anchor point.
2. Get into an athletic stance and press the cable or band straight out in front of you *(a)*.
3. Your arms and the cable or band should form a 90-degree angle so that you feel a rotational force through your hips and torso.

EXECUTION

1. Hold the setup position if the set is timed.
2. If the set is for repetitions, bring your hands into your chest *(b)* and press back out to the beginning position.
3. Manual resistance can be applied in the absence of a band or cable.

HALF KNEELING CHOP AND LIFT

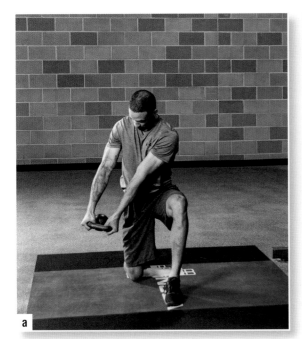
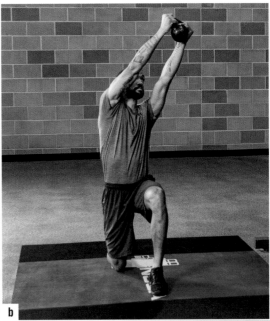

SETUP

1. Assume a tall half kneeling position with your front and rear knees both forming a 90-degree angle.

2. Your feet should be in line with your hips or narrower.

3. Hold a weight in your hands with your arms extended.

VARIATION SETUP

If using a band, anchor it low and to your side of the down leg to load the lift portion, or anchor it high and to the side of the up leg to load the chop portion of the exercise.

EXECUTION

1. Begin with the weight next to your pocket on the side of the down knee *(a)*. Bring the weight across your body and up in a diagonal fashion, rotating through your upper back *(b)*.

2. Control the range of motion, and bring the weight back down to where it started.

VARIATION EXECUTION

If using a band, it will provide resistance during either the chop or the lift, so consider doing repetitions with both a chop emphasis and a lift emphasis for each set.

COMMON FAULT

■ *Losing positional integrity.* Keep the arms long and stay tall through your hips and torso while moving through a controlled range of motion.

STIR THE POT

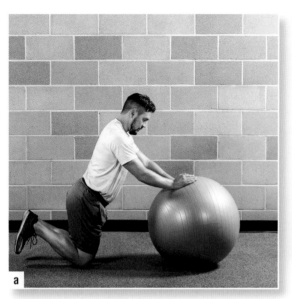
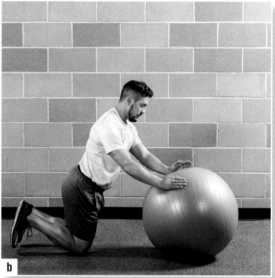

SETUP

1. Start in a tall kneeling position, forming a straight line from your knees through the top of your head.

2. Keep your arms straight and place your hands on the piece of equipment being used (e.g., roller, stability ball *[a]*, suspension trainer).

EXECUTION

1. Fall forward slightly to achieve increased tension in your abdominals while maintaining a straight line from your head through your knees.

2. Keep your torso and lower body still and your arms long while moving your hands and arms in small circles as if stirring a giant pot of stew *(b)*.

COMMON FAULT

- *Breaking at the hips.* Resist the urge to let your butt kick backward and lose the straight line from your head to your knees. You should feel tension in your abdominals through the whole exercise. It helps to move slower than you think you want to.

ROMAN SIDE CRUNCH

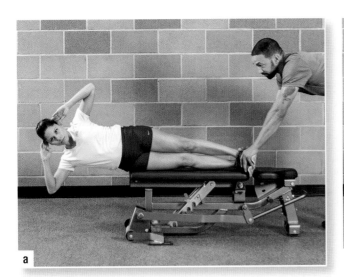 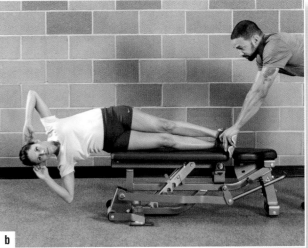

SETUP

1. Lie laterally on a glute ham or Roman chair bench. Alternatively, you can lie laterally on a flat bench with a partner holding your legs down.

2. Your hips should be in contact with the bench, but your oblique abdominals and upper body should be unsupported.

3. Your body should be in a straight line from the head to the heel. This is the beginning position *(a)*.

EXECUTION

1. From the beginning position, laterally flex at the hip as if doing a side bend *(b)*.

2. Once you have flexed maximally (range of motion will vary), return to the beginning position.

3. To add weight, you can hold the weight against your chest.

COMMON FAULT

■ *Using momentum to achieve range of motion.* Slow the movement down to a point where you can stop at any moment throughout the range of motion. If this is not possible, consider substituting a side plank, single-arm farmer walk, or dumbbell side bend.

BODY SAW

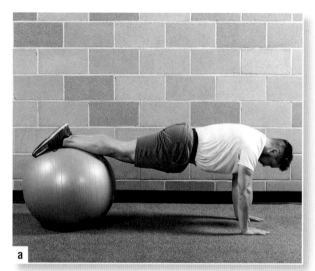
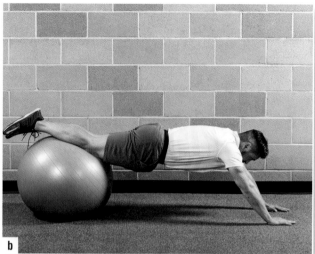

SETUP

1. Start in a front plank position with your toes on a pair of sliders or suspension trainer (6 inches [15 cm] off the floor).

2. If you have a stability ball, you can perform the exercise with your arms extended as in the top of a push-up and your toes supported by the ball *(a)*.

EXECUTION

1. Maintaining the plank position, drive forward through your elbows and forearms to push your body backward, increasing the tension on your abdominals.

2. Push as far back as possible without compromising positional integrity *(b)*.

3. Pull through the elbows and forearms to return to the beginning position.

COMMON FAULTS

■ *Hips sagging.* Pull your hips off the floor so that your body is in a straight line and you feel the exercise in the front of your body and not your lower back.

■ *Hips going too high.* Squeeze your butt to straighten your hips and keep a straight line from your head to your heels.

SIDE BEND

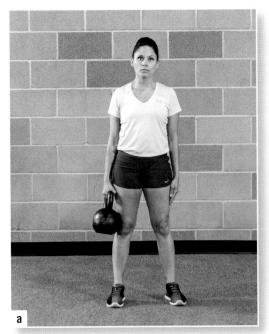

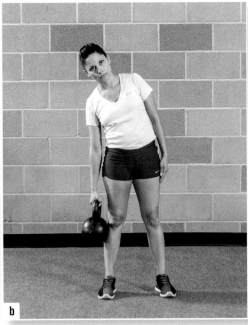

SETUP

Stand tall with a dumbbell at your side and your arm straight *(a)*.

VARIATION SETUP

If using a band, loop it under one foot and grasp the free running end with the same side hand, choking up as much as needed to achieve sufficient resistance.

EXECUTION

1. Push your hips in the opposite direction of the dumbbell and allow the upper back to flex laterally so the dumbbell travels slightly down the side of your body *(b)*.

2. Reverse course to return to the start position.

FARMER WALK

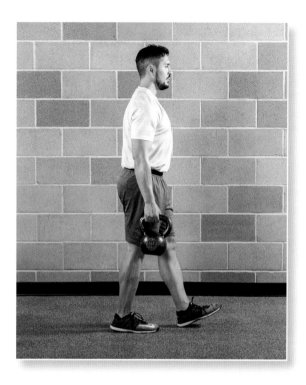

SETUP

1. Stand tall and hold a dumbbell or kettlebell in each hand while keeping your arms long.

2. If performing the exercise with a single arm, keep your body's alignment integrity intact as if you were holding a weight in each hand.

EXECUTION

Maintain your tall posture while walking (not running) smoothly for the assigned distance.

COMMON FAULTS

■ *Bending the arms.* Keep your arms straight, and do not let the weight rest on your legs while you walk. Do not shrug.

■ *Bending over.* Maintain a tall position throughout the walk.

■ *Choosing incorrect weight.* Select a weight that challenges you for the duration but that you do not need to set down before completion.

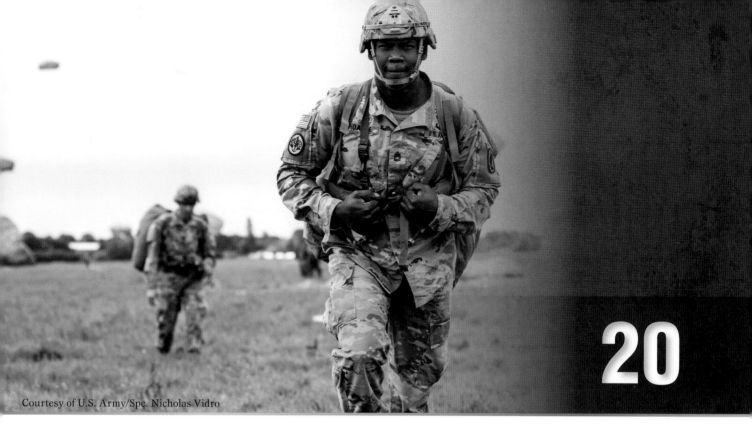

Courtesy of U.S. Army/Spc. Nicholas Vidro

Conditioning

Traditionally, the intensity of conditioning sessions has been measured by the amount of sweat expired or the distance covered. Rather than relying solely on volume, the conditioning prescriptions within this ACFT training program purposefully manipulate volume, intensity, and exercise type. Doing so yields an efficient, effective dose that causes adaptations to improve performance on the SDC and 2MR while also improving recoverability between all ACFT events. Follow the objective and subjective intensity guidelines to achieve the desired outcome of each conditioning protocol. This likely means working both harder and easier, at times, than you are used to, but it is important that you trust the program. Abandon your comfort zone by pushing harder for some shorter duration activities and holding back on some longer duration activities.

Sometimes you do not have access to the assigned equipment for a particular exercise nor space to run for running-based conditioning workouts. In these instances, intelligently selected alternatives can still move the conditioning needle in the right direction. Each exercise has three obvious components: distance or duration, intensity, and specificity. When choosing a substitute exercise, try to match each of these as closely as possible to mimic the exercise's intended physical demands. Substitutes are often obvious but other times require some creativity. However, lack of equipment or space should never serve as an excuse to completely abandon the prescribed conditioning. When possible, consult a certified coach to learn about an appropriate alternative for both strength and conditioning exercises.

50, 100, AND 150 YARD SHUTTLES

Perform shuttles on a surface that allows safe change of direction. Start in a split stance position or prone position. Sprint 25 yards (23 m) as fast as possible, decelerating and changing direction as efficiently as possible to sprint back toward the start. Continue this process until you cover the total prescribed distance. Rest for the advised amount of time before completing subsequent repetitions. Each repetition should be performed at maximum speed.

400 METER, 800 METER, AND ONE MILE REPEATS

A track is preferred for repeats, but you can use a treadmill or any measured course that allows for continuous running. For these exercises, it is extremely important to adhere to the prescribed pace and rest periods. During some sessions the pace is faster than your two-mile pace and therefore provides speed training. Other sessions might be equal to or slower than your two-mile pace and therefore intends to accumulate volume at submaximal speeds. Sometimes your rest is prescribed in a work-to-rest (W:R) ratio, which expresses how long you should rest compared to how long it takes you to complete the work. For example, a 1:1 W:R ratio means to rest for the same amount of time it takes to complete the repetition. If you completed a 400-meter (440 yd) run in 60 seconds, then you rest for 60 seconds.

THREE TO FIVE MILE RUN AND FIVE TO SIX MILE RUCK

Runs and rucks for distance are common in traditional military training. While the program intends to reduce the running volumes typically included within PT, these are still an effective way to build capacity while incorporating specificity. The ruck is less specific to the ACFT but still specific to soldiering, so it is also included as an option for building capacity. These runs and rucks should be performed at a steady pace. Once you have found your groove, limit variability in intensity and pace. These should be performed fast enough that you can only string together one or two consecutive sentences. If you are unable to do so, you are going too fast; if you can hold a continuous conversation, you are going too slow.

A more precise tool to monitor intensity during training is exercise heart rate which is based on a percent of maximum heart rate (MHR). A simple formula to estimate MHR is 220 – age (e.g., if you are 20 years old, your MHR is 200 beats per minute). Commonly, exercise heart rate is targeted to be between 70 percent and 80 percent or 75 percent and 85 percent of MHR.

40 YARD BUILD-UPS

This simple drill serves as a warm-up specific to running. Start the drill in a staggered stance. Accelerate slowly and change gears to gradually increase speed about every 10 yards (9 m) until you cover a distance of 40 yards (37 m). Run through the finish line and gradually decelerate instead of coming to a sudden stop. You should increase speed smoothly with your knees driving a little higher as speed increases. These will always be performed for multiple repetitions. Finish the first repetition at about 70 percent of your maximum speed and the last repetition at maximal or near maximal speed. You are not only gradually increasing speed within each repetition, but from repetition to repetition.

FAN BIKE INTERVALS

Sitting on a fan bike with a seat height that allows for a slight bend in the knee when the pedal is in the bottom position, sprint as fast as possible for the assigned duration, distance, or caloric expenditure. These intervals must be performed at an all-out effort.

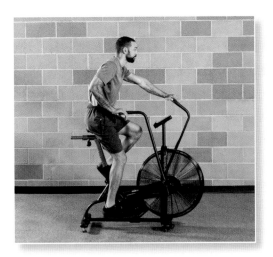

ROW ERGOMETER

When rowing on an ergometer (often shortened to *rower*), you should sequentially but seamlessly extend first your knees, then your hips, and finish the repetition by rowing toward your chest with the upper body. To return to the start position, perform the reverse actions in the reverse order by extending your arms and then by flexing your hips and knees. A resistance damper setting of 5 to 7 is recommended, but a stronger individual might prefer a higher setting while a weaker individual might prefer a lower setting. Maintain the same setting for all repetitions for comparative performance purposes.

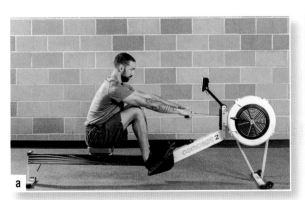
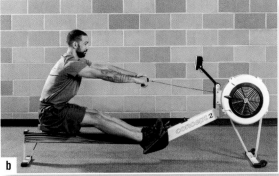
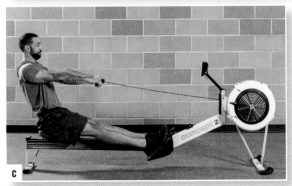
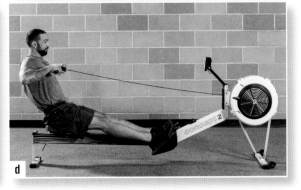

TIME TRIAL

Cover the assigned distance as fast as possible using the designated type of exercise, and rest for the prescribed time. Compete against yourself or other soldiers to meet the intent of an all-out effort.

15-MINUTE TIMED BLOCK – SLED PUSH AND DUMBBELL FARMER WALK

This conditioning session is simple but has a high-density workload. Load a sled up heavy enough that you cannot easily run with it and grab a pair of heavy dumbbells. Push the sled down and back 15 yards (14 m). Pick up (without straps) the dumbbells and walk tall (do not run) down and back the same 15 yards (14 m), keeping your arms straight. Set the dumbbells down without dropping them. You have now completed one round. Complete as many rounds as possible within the 15-minute time block. If you are able to finish more than 10 rounds within the 15-minute block, increase the weights next session. Your farmer walk weight is often limited by grip strength, so increase the weight on the sled once grip is the limiting factor.

EVERY MINUTE ON THE MINUTE (EMOM) CIRCUITS

EMOM circuits provide a creative means of accumulating total work while practicing exercises in small doses. At the top of each minute, perform the prescribed circuit in its entirety and then rest for the remainder of the minute. Performing five push-ups in succession is a small task, but you will accumulate 100 repetitions within a 20-minute EMOM circuit. If you cannot perform the assigned number of repetitions in unbroken succession, substitute an assisted or easier version. You should not rest between repetitions.

ROUNDS FOR TIME

Rounds for time are fairly intuitive. Perform the prescribed exercises for the repetitions, distance, or calories assigned as a paired set or circuit for the total number of rounds provided in as little time as possible. Rest as little as possible, if at all, within the session. These sessions often pair unrelated exercises to minimize localized muscle fatigue and maximize intensity. Rounds for time serve as a great challenge or competitive undertaking.

BACKWARD SLED DRAG + SHUTTLES

Load a sled with 90 pounds (41 kg), the same weight as the SDC event. Drag the sled backward 25 yards (23 m) down and back as fast as possible. Once you drag the sled past the start line, immediately drop the straps and sprint the same 25 yards (23 m) down and back. Repeat for the assigned number of repetitions, resting for the prescribed amount of time. In the absence of a sled, running backward uphill can provide a similar overload.

ACRONYMS AND ABBREVIATIONS

1RM: one repetition maximum

2MR: Two-Mile Run

a: acceleration

ACFT: Army Combat Fitness Test

Alt: alternating

AMRAP: as many repetitions as possible

APFT: Army Physical Fitness Test

BB: barbell

BMI: body mass index

DB: dumbbell

ECC: eccentric emphasis

EMOM: every minute on the minute

F: force

HRP: Hand Release Push-Up–Arm Extension

ISO: isometric

KB: kettlebell

LTK: Leg Tuck

m: mass

MB: medicine ball

MDL: 3 Repetition Maximum Deadlift

METL: mission essential task listings

MHR: maximum heart rate

MOS: military occupational specialties

MR: multiple response

MWR: Morale, Welfare, and Recreation

P: power

PT: physical training

RDL: Romanian deadlift

RFE: rear foot elevated

RG: reverse grip

SA: single arm

SB: stability ball

SDC: Sprint-Drag-Carry

SL: single leg

SR: single response

SPT: Standing Power Throw

TAP-C: Tactical Athlete Performance Center

v: velocity

W:R ratio: work-to-rest ratio

WTBD: warrior tasks and battle drills

Wtd: weighted

GLOSSARY

absolute strength—How much total force you can apply maximally for one repetition.

aerobic endurance—The ability to perform long-duration activities at a high steady state; supports your ability to recover between events.

agility—Similar to speed—acceleration, maintenance of continuous (often top-end) speed, and deceleration—but executed multidirectionally.

anaerobic endurance—The ability to produce a specific amount of work in the shortest amount of time possible.

athleticism—The ability to dynamically transition between positions.

body composition—What the body is made of and is typically associated with fat mass and fat-free mass.

coordination—*See* athleticism.

core—Also called the trunk of the body.

duration—How long you train.

flexibility—The ability of a muscle to stretch.

frequency—How often you train.

individuality—The quality of one person being different from another.

movement competency—The ability to achieve the positions and rhythm necessary to coordinate movement without compensatory patterns.

muscular endurance—The ability to repeatedly move a submaximal load for a given number of repetitions or time, as well as an extended amount of time.

muscular strength—An expression of how much force can be applied to move an external object or one's own mass.

one-repetition maximum—The maximal force you can apply for one repetition.

overload—Adjustment of the intensity, volume, or complexity of an exercise to force your body to adapt favorably.

power—An expression of force times velocity ($P = F \times v$).

progression—The continued application of overload.

readiness—The ability to meet the physical demands of any combat or duty position, accomplish the mission, and continue to fight and win.

relative strength—How strong you are compared to your body weight.

specificity—The principle of targeting physical characteristics related to those present in the successful execution of the ACFT or your job.

speed—Acceleration, maintenance of continuous (often top-end) speed, and deceleration, all occurring in a linear fashion.

triple extension—Extension (straightening) of the ankles, knees, and hips.

SUGGESTED RESOURCES

Alvar, BA, Sell, K, and Deuster, PA, eds. *NSCA's Essentials of Tactical Strength and Conditioning.* Champaign, IL: Human Kinetics, 2017.

Barringer, N, Rooney, M. The rush: How speed can save lives. *Infantry*, April-July 2016. www.benning.army.mil/Infantry/Magazine/issues/2016/APR-JUL/pdf/4)%20Barringer_Rush.pdf.

Barringer, N, Rooney, M. What is the rush? NSCA TSAC conference, Orlando, FL, April 2017.

Clark, N. *Nancy Clark's Sports Nutrition Guidebook.* 6th ed. Champaign, IL: Human Kinetics, 2020.

Dawes, J. *Complete Guide to TRX Suspension Training.* Champaign, IL: Human Kinetics, 2017.

de la Motte, SJ, Lisman, P, Sabatino, M, Beutler, AI, O'Connor, FG, Deuster, PA. The relationship between functional movement, balance deficits, and previous injury history in deploying marine warfighters. *Journal of Strength and Conditioning Research*, 30(6):1619-1625, 2016.

East, WB. *A historical review and analysis of Army physical readiness training and assessment.* Army Command and General Staff College Fort Leavenworth KS Combat Studies Institute, 2013. https://apps.dtic.mil/dtic/tr/fulltext/u2/a622014.pdf. Accessed March 11, 2020.

EXOS. EXOS presents tactical training systems. Accessed March 19, 2020. www.teamexos.com/exos-presents-tactical.

INSEP, Hausswirth, C and Mujika, I, eds. *Recovery for Performance in Sport.* Champaign, IL: Human Kinetics, 2013.

Kellman, M, and Beckman, J, eds. *Sport, Recovery, and Performance: Interdisciplinary Insights.* Oxon, UK: Routledge, 2018.

Kelso, T. *The Interval Training Manual: 520+ Interval Running Workouts for All Sports and Abilities.* Monterey, CA: Coaches Choice, 2005.

Knapik, JJ, and East, WB. History of United States Army Physical Fitness and physical readiness testing. *US Army Medical Department Journal* 5-19, 2014.

Knapik, JJ, Redmond, JE, Grier, TL, and Sharp, MA. Secular trends in the physical fitness of United States Army infantry units and infantry soldiers, 1976–2015. *Military Medicine* 183(11-12):e414-e426, 2018.

National Strength and Conditioning Association. National Strength and Conditioning Association's tactical annual training conference. Accessed March 19, 2020. www.nsca.com/events/conferences/tactical-training.

National Strength and Conditioning Association. National Strength and Conditioning Association's tactical strength and conditioning course. Accessed March 19, 2020. www.nsca.com/education/courses/tsac-practitioners-course.

National Strength and Conditioning Association. *TSAC Report.* Accessed March 19, 2020. www.nsca.com/education/journals/tsac-report.

O2X Human Performance. Accessed March 19, 2020. https://o2x.com.

O2X Human Performance. *Human Performance for Tactical Athletes.* Tulsa, OK: Fire Engineering Books, 2019.

Palkoska, F. *Army Physical Fitness Update: Training the Tactical Athlete for the Army of 2025.* U.S. Army Physical Fitness School, 2015.

Roy, TC, Lopez, HP, Piva, SR. Loads worn by soldiers predict episodes of low back pain during deployment to Afghanistan. *Spine*, 38(15):1310-1317, 2013.

Schierberl, C, Bigham, D. *How to Build the Tactical Athlete for the United States Army.* Tactical Athlete Performance Training Center, 2016.

United States Army. Army Combat Fitness Test. Accessed March 19, 2020. www.army.mil/acft.

United States Army. Army Combat Fitness Test FY20 standards. Accessed March 19, 2020. www.army.mil/e2/downloads/rv7/acft/fy20_standards.pdf.

United States Army. *FM 7-22: Army Physical Readiness Training.* Accessed March 19, 2020. https://armypubs.army.mil/epubs/DR_pubs/DR_a/pdf/web/ARN7938_FM%207-22%20INC%20C1%20Final.pdf.

United States Army, Combined Arms Center. The human dimension white paper: A framework for optimizing human performance. October 9, 2014. Accessed March 11, 2020. http://usacac.army.mil/sites/default/files/documents/cact/HumanDimensionWhitePaper.pdf.

Volt Athletics. Accessed March 19, 2020. www.voltathletics.com.

ABOUT THE NSCA

Founded in 1978, The National Strength and Conditioning Association (NSCA) is a nonprofit association dedicated to advancing the strength and conditioning and related sport science professions around the world.

The NSCA exists to empower a community of professionals to maximize their impact through disseminating evidence-based knowledge and its practical application by offering industry-leading certifications, research journals, career development services, networking opportunities, and continuing education. The NSCA community is composed of more than 60,000 members and certified professionals throughout the world who further industry standards as researchers, educators, strength and conditioning coaches, performance and sport scientists, personal trainers, tactical professionals, and other related roles.

Nate Palin, MS, CSCS, is the tactical strength and conditioning program manager for the National Strength and Conditioning Association (NSCA). Prior to his transition to the strength and conditioning profession, he served as a leader in the 2nd Ranger Battalion for seven years. Over the course of five combat deployments in support of Operation Enduring Freedom and Operation Iraqi Freedom, Palin experienced the military's performance shortcomings and observed the need for enhanced physical training to better support mission critical tasks. These experiences drove him to begin his coaching career in 2010, narrowing his focus to tactical strength and conditioning as a performance specialist for EXOS in Washington, D.C., in 2012. He coached Special Operations Forces at Joint Base Lewis-McChord from 2015 to 2018.

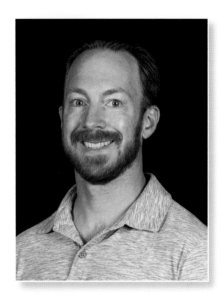

Rob Hartman, MAEd, CSCS, serves as a strength and conditioning professional who is contracted to implement, analyze, and guide numerous aspects of the Special Operations Human Performance Program at the unit level. He began his career servicing the Special Operations community in late 2010, spending the first six years with the 1st Special Forces Group and more recent years working with the Special Operations Aviation Regiment.

During his tenure in the tactical community, Hartman educated others in the field with his participation in the NSCA's TSAC Practitioners Course, EXOS' Tactical Training course, NSCA's TSAC Annual Training conference, the Tactical Athlete Human Factors Summit, and briefs to various units on Joint Base Lewis-McChord. His experience allows him to be consulted for macro and micro areas in the field, but he typically deals with modeling programming and profiling of tactical operators' aerobic and anaerobic attributes.

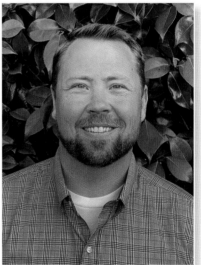

Photo courtesy of Shannon Hartman.

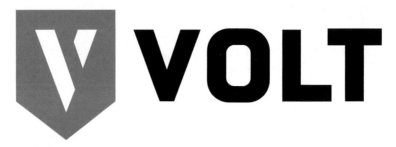

Volt Athletics teamed up with Human Kinetics to create an app based on the training programs included in chapter 12 of this book to help you prepare for the Army Combat Fitness Test!

To unlock the ACFT Prep program using a promo code that provides <u>30% off standard subscription rates</u>, follow the steps below.

Step 1: On your mobile phone, go to https://volt.app/ACFTprep. The promo code of HKACFT will appear in the first field. Enter your email address and click "Apply Code."

Step 2: You should see a message that says, "Promo code applied!" On this screen, enter your name, date of birth, and a password for your account. Tap "Create Account."

Step 3: You should see a message that says, "Your Volt account has been created!" Tap the link to download the Volt app from your phone's app store.

Step 4: After downloading the Volt app, tap the white "<u>Log in to your account</u>" button and enter your email address and the password you created in Step 2. Then, follow the screen prompts to fully personalize your ACFT prep program!

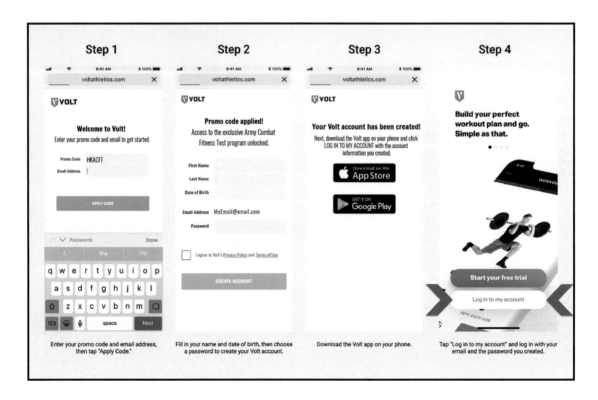

Please email support@voltathletics.com with any questions about setting up or using your Volt account.

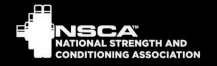
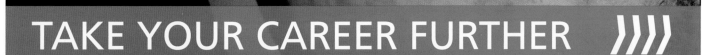
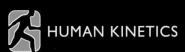

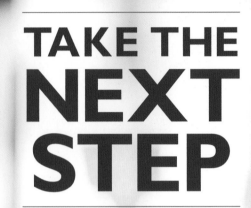

TAKE THE
NEXT
STEP

A continuing education course
is available for this text.
Find out more.

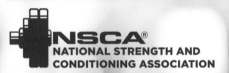

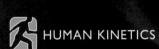